MW01295973

Forgetting How to Remember

Alzheimer's disease: a modern plague with staggering implications for human mental health

Vincent T Marchesi MD PhD
Professor of Pathology`
Yale University
vincent.marchesi@yale.edu

VINCENT T MARCHESI

Copyright © 2019 Vincent T. Marchesi
All rights reserved.

ISBN: 9781796462067

DEDICATION

For Sally Lockwood Marchesi, who provided the energy and the inspiration for an entire family

CONTENTS

ACKNOWLEDGMENTS

Many people have been involved in the production of this book. Special thanks for editorial assistance provided by Steve Vance and members of my family and close friends including Sarah and Julia Marchesi, Andrea Thais, and Kevin Callahan.

Support for the studies that led to this work was provided by the Anthony N. Brady endowment of Yale University

CHAPTER 1

HOW IT BEGAN

On a crisp fall day in September, 1953 Henry Molaison, known to psychologists as H.M., underwent a surgical operation that changed his life forever. After a prolonged operation at the Hartford Hospital in Hartford Connecticut, he awoke groggy but in good spirits. When visited by his surgeon and members of the nursing staff he seemed alert and cooperative but said little. The next day the same team came by for a second visit and asked the same questions. Henry had no idea who they were, and he asked where he was and why he was there. He was relieved and greatly pleased when his parents entered his hospital room. They explained to him that he had had an operation that was meant to relieve him of the repeated seizures that had made his life unbearable. He seemed pleased to learn that he would be free of those horrible seizures that he suffered throughout his life. The next day when his parents returned, he asked them again why he was in the hospital. It soon became apparent that Henry had no memory of what they said the day before. Most remarkably, Henry was unable to remember any new thought or experience for more than few minutes after it happened, yet he could recall many aspects of his life that happened before the operation. This inability to remember the recent past also made it difficult for him to anticipate what might happen in the future.

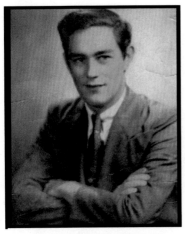

Henry Molaison (H.M.)
(1926-2008)

H.M. often referred to as the man who lost his ability to remember new things became highly sought-after by psychologists and neuroscientists, each hoping he might provide insights into the mechanisms of memory[1] He was described as a friendly cooperative subject who seemed to enjoy being studied and found each test a new experience no matter how many times he had been exposed to it. He lived to be eighty-two years old and died in 2008. But this operation, tragic as it was for H.M., led to an avalanche of studies on the mechanism of human memory. Before this fateful operation it was assumed that memory functions were scattered throughout the brain, but since Dr. Scoville had only removed small portions of what are called the temporal lobes that included the hippocampus[2] it was realized and subsequently confirmed that part of our ability to remember recent events was largely confined to this part of the brain.

This discovery had many practical consequences. It led investigators to look for the cause of dementia first by autopsy studies and later by magnetic resonance studies (MRI) of living patients[3].The operation undertaken to reduce epileptic seizures provided dramatic proof that one particular part of the brain known as the hippocampus was an important memory center.

Overview

Alzheimer's dementia[4], its causes and what we can do about it have been the subject of intense scientific investigation for more than four decades. There are many possible causes of this complex disease, among the most talked about are mysterious protein deposits[5] called amyloid[6] and tau[7] that were first described more than a century ago, but these are only two of many possible causes of brain damage that lead to dementia.

As is true of any study of a human disease, investigators working in the Alzheimer's field have focused primarily on disease processes that physically damage the brain, assuming that mental impairment must be caused by a recognizable disease. But during the last half decade a new idea has emerged. We are now asking the question: does the intact undamaged brain itself contribute to mental impairment? A strong case can be made that an inactive brain, like an inactive muscle, runs the risk of losing its capacity to function properly. Muscles that are challenged by exercise increase their size and strength, but muscles that remain inactive for long periods of time shrink down due to a process called disuse atrophy. The brain, it turns out, behaves very much like a muscle. After the normal growth period of the brain, which extends through the mid-20s of human life, the brain only grows in response to challenges that are imposed upon it. The prolonged absence of challenging mental activities leads to reduced capacity.

Studies of the lifestyles of elderly people turn out to be very revealing. What they eat, how they exercise, and how they think have become of great concern since these factors affect both their likelihood to develop both cardiovascular disease and impaired mental status in later life. Physical exercise increases one's mental capacity by supplying more blood to the brain and by activating factors that can affect the growth and ability of nerve cells to connect with each other. Challenging mental activities behave similarly. And the degree of challenge turns out to be just as important. In order for the brain to grow it must learn something new, and this learning process must be incremental. Learning a new language, learning how to play a musical instrument, or other challenging mental exercises clearly have a positive impact. People who have been involved with demanding activities during their adult years clearly benefit from the challenges that their brains have experienced. But retirement changes all that. Occupational challenges are lost, and, unless they are replaced by other demanding intellectual activities, the inactive brain gradually loses its edge.

Proposing that early dementia involves impaired functions of the brain that are reversible is a positive prospect, since it implies that if we understand how brain functions are impaired and learn how to block their action, we can reverse the problems of many people who are still in the early stages of what could be a reversible problem. The conclusion to be drawn from these new studies is that Alzheimer's disease (abbreviated as AD) has many causes, some known but many others still to be identified. Because of these gaps in our knowledge, focusing on treatments designed to attack specific causes have so far been largely ineffective. Indeed, it is ironic that we live in an era of biomedical advances that are truly revolutionary, yet the only FDA approved treatment for Alzheimer's dementia now available was discovered more than 30 years ago.

What have proved to be effective are preventive measures based on the practices of people who reach late adulthood with intact cognitive abilities. The good news is that the adult human brain can be a work in progress if appropriate measures are taken to nourish it and train it. Diseases do indeed damage the brain and account for a large fraction of people afflicted with dementia, but it is now clear that a significant number of people at risk can be rescued by appropriate preventive measures. Indeed, recent studies show that the incidence of dementia is actually decreasing significantly (approximately 25%) in populations who are practicing what are perceived to be protective measures [8] even though the total number of people who have the disease is increasing as populations age.

The Beginning

The story of this terrible malady known as Alzheimer's dementia (AD) that now affects millions of aging people was first revealed on November 4, 1906 at a meeting of German psychiatrists in Tubingen, Germany by Alois Alzheimer. He described a 51-year-old woman who was suffering from an incapacitating loss of memory and violent hallucinations that eventually led to her inability to communicate.

Auguste Deter was born on May 16, 1850, in Cassel Germany and died on April 8, 1906, 55 years later. Five years before her death she developed a strange set of symptoms that became increasingly alarming to her railway worker husband. These included a bizarre series of hallucinations. She became fearful that people were trying to kill her and even accused her husband of being unfaithful. Her inability to remember things became progressively worse, as did her abilities to read and write. At night unable to sleep, she would often drag sheets throughout the house for hours while screaming. She eventually lost the ability to care for herself, and her husband was forced to hospitalize her in the Community Psychiatric Hospital at Frankfurt am Main, on Nov 26, 1901. There she encountered for the first time Dr. Alois Alzheimer, a psychiatrist specializing in mental disorders.

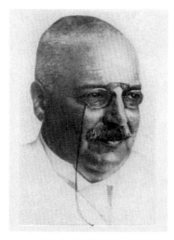

**Alois Alzheimer
(1864-1915)**

Alzheimer found her very puzzling. She had all the symptoms and characteristics of someone suffering from advanced dementia, but at age 51 she was at least two decades younger than the usual patient with that condition. After she died in 1906, Alzheimer had the chance to examine her brain after an autopsy. What he found was most surprising. Deposits of material he had never seen before were scattered throughout her brain. He described them as either irregular shaped aggregates that occupied spaces between the brain cells or string-like forms that were embedded within the cells themselves. He called the clumped material plaques and the string-like forms tangles. Alzheimer had no idea what these deposits were, nor could he explain how they might have caused her behavior. It was not possible in 1906 to find out what plaques and tangles were. Indeed, it would take sixty years of advanced basic science research to answer these questions. But Alzheimer's discovery of these plaques and tangles (terms still in use today) was the first step in defining and hopefully explaining the mental condition that we call Alzheimer's disease.

The idea that brain damage might be caused by the accumulation of a toxic substance was a new idea and a very important one, since it provided for the first time a source of damage to the brain that had never been observed before. It was in many ways a great breakthrough since it now provided a target to focus on. Instead of assuming that the brains of old people were simply wearing out as was the assumption at that time, it was now possible to think that brains of mentally impaired people were damaged by specific toxic substances. If indeed toxic substances were accumulating in the brains of people as they aged, they would be potential therapeutic targets. Knowing a cause of a disease has always been the surest way to the development of an effective treatment. Unfortunately, the scientific tools needed to isolate and characterize these unknown deposits had not yet been invented, so the chemical nature of them remained unknown for eighty years.

Memory Loss

The most characteristic feature of Alzheimer's dementia is memory loss. All of us who have family members or close friends who are in the early stages of dementia witness what we call forgetfulness or the inability to remember things that happened a few minutes before. While loss of memory is a common complaint of senior people it is certainly not an inevitable sign of impending dementia. We now realize there are many reasons why people forget things. In fact, the ability of the brain to forget is just as important as its ability to remember. The human brain has the remarkable capacity to acquire, store, and eventually recall massive amounts of information, some of which can persist in the brain over decades of time. Not only does the brain have what appears to be an inexhaustible capacity to retain information, it must also have an extremely effective memory management system, since retrieval of memories is seamless, rapid, and remarkably efficient. Another important feature of our brains is the ability to remove memories that are no longer useful. Some psychologists even believe that we have the ability to actively forget memories that evoke guilt or embarrassment. For all these reasons the inability to remember things often has nothing at all to do with the development of dementia.

Most of the memories that we experience last for a very short time usually seconds or minutes. These are called short-term memories, and loss of them is one of the most characteristic features of the early stages of Alzheimer's dementia. Another set of memories can last for hours and days, and yet still another set can last for decades. These long-term memories are often the last to be lost during the last stages of dementia.

Memories can also play tricks on themselves. Some memories cancel out the ability to store new ones while other memories can block the capacity to retrieve previously stored ones[9]. These mechanisms of interference are not understood, but they are an important feature of everyday working memory. There is a general consensus that sleep enhances the process of memory consolidation leading to enhanced memory expression after sleep. But there is also an alternative view that sleep suppresses forgetting. It is possible that sleep can affect memory through enhanced consolidation or the combined efforts of reduced forgetting and the blocking of interference factors.

Alzheimer's discovery of potentially toxic material in impaired brains was novel and interesting, but it raised an important question: how could such deposits affect a person's ability to remember? The prevailing view (based more on speculation than scientific fact) was that memories were created and stored over the entire part of the brain called the cerebral cortex [10]. Yet the deposits he described were often localized to specific parts of the brain, which made it difficult to understand how they were able to damage all the memory centers of the brain that were scattered throughout the entire cortex.

CHAPTER 2

SEARCH FOR A CAUSE

In modern times, as was true in the past, many catastrophic illnesses were prevented when their causes were determined. Treatments of polio and AIDS are two examples of triumphs of medical science that happened during our lifetimes. Both were achieved when their causes were identified. In each case an infectious agent was the culprit, and modern science was used to eradicate its affects. It is important to realize that each of these problems had a single cause and once this was identified successful treatments could be devised.

As far as we can tell, dementia and its accompanying impairments have afflicted human beings for as long as they were able to live long enough to develop them. This is not to say that dementia is the inevitable consequence of growing old or even the result of the aging process. Mental impairments result from many causes, some beginning long before the signs of dementia become evident, and many of them take time to develop into serious consequences. Present estimates suggest that the beginning stages of the disease begin 20 or more years before symptoms are evident. Before Alzheimer's discovery there was no reason to suspect that toxic material might be the cause of dementia. Indeed, it was widely believed that the brain was simply wearing out or growing old, explanations that were neither scientifically accurate nor helpful in determining causation.

The Amyloid Hypothesis [11]

For many decades Alzheimer's discovery had little impact on our understanding of dementia. Other scientists repeated his observations, but there was no way to relate their findings to the cause of the disease. Simply looking at brains with advanced disease after autopsy analysis gave little insight into the processes that were responsible for the various clinical problems. It was not until the 1960s that neuroscientists began to re-examine the mysterious deposits that Alzheimer described using more modern tools including the electron microscope. When examined with this powerful new microscope the deposits appeared to be bundles of strand-like material referred to as fibrils, but even then it was not possible to identify their chemical nature, nor was there any universal agreement that these fibrils were in any way related to the cause of dementia.

There was little progress in identifying the chemical nature of the material Alzheimer described until George Glenner, an American pathologist working at the National Institutes of Health in the 1980s, made the decisive breakthrough. [12]

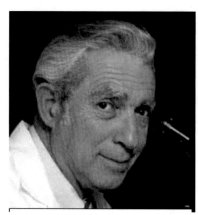

**George Glenner
(1928-1995)**

As is so often the case with major discoveries in medical research, Glenner was not working on dementia at the time. His focus was on a disease called amyloidosis, which also involved deposits of unknown material in major organs of the body that inevitably led to heart failure and death. Because amyloidosis also affects blood vessels, Glenner extracted material from blood vessels obtained from brains of deceased Alzheimer's patients using modern biochemical techniques that were not available to Alzheimer. To his surprise he found that the mysterious deposits that Alzheimer described were composed of fragments of the body's own protein molecules. This stunning discovery ignited a firestorm of investigation of this intriguing material (called amyloid) throughout the world. Laboratories in

Germany, Australia, and Brooklyn (NY) came to the same conclusion; amyloid was made up of digestion products of a protein molecule that was needed for normal brain function[13].

Modern DNA technology made it possible to identify the gene that produces the amyloid peptides. [14] After this discovery the search was on to find out whether the gene was abnormal in people with dementia. Alison Goate and a team of coworkers at St Mary's Hospital Medical School in London studied eleven families that had many members afflicted with dementia. By comparing the genes in each family, a single mutation was detected that was only present in the family members who had dementia. This finding, reported in 1991, was quickly confirmed and extended by other investigators throughout the world.

A similar mutation was found in thousands of affected people living in the small village of Medellin in Colombia, South America. They were suffering from an especially debilitating form of dementia that had all the earmarks of a 14th century plague. When a disease affects so many people in a community as this one seemed to be doing, some infectious process is almost always discovered. Rodent-borne bacteria spread the bubonic plague in northern Italy in 1360s, and in more recent times viral influenza killed millions of Americans in 1918. Could the dementia of these Colombians be due to some unknown infectious agent?

Thankfully, for them and the rest of us, the answer is most definitely no. After lengthy investigations their problem was found to have a distinct genetic basis. Because they lived in an isolated region in the Andes mountains for seven generations and intermarried, everyone in the village was related to a man who migrated from Spain in the 17th century and settled there. This unknown individual had the capacity to transmit to his descendants a genetic mutation that has the potential to cause severe dementia and progressive memory loss in those who inherit it. This was truly a genetic curse, but not the only one. There are other equally devastating genes, fortunately very rare, that also guarantee that the bearer of a mutation will develop early onset dementia. The link between these mutations and disease soon became apparent when it was discovered that they enhanced the production of amyloid. This convinced many investigators that amyloid was the cause of the dementia and led many to conclude that Alzheimer's dementia was an inherited disease.

But soon the story became more complicated. As more people who suffered from dementia were studied it became apparent that most people with dementia do not have the types of defective genes that Goate and others had discovered. Since people with defective genes developed problems earlier than those lacking them, their condition was described as early onset. Affected people who do not have these genes (95% of affected patients) are considered to have late onset dementia. Later studies revealed that they were subject to another potential genetic pitfall that is much more prevalent, the ApoE protein now the subject of intense study and much speculation[15].

The deposits that Alzheimer called plaques turned out to be accumulations of amyloid that clumped together around the nerve cells and the structures he called tangles were composed of another protein, called tau, that formed clumps inside nerve cells. Both were often accompanied by the loss of brain cells in advanced stages of disease. Since brain cell death was considered the point of no return, the three together, plaques, tangles, and dead cells, were considered by many investigators to be the obvious cause of dementia.

The Brain Scan: a diagnostic break through

For years the autopsy remained the only reliable way to decide whether individuals with signs of dementia really had amyloid plaques in their brains. This changed dramatically when investigators at the University of Pittsburgh developed a way to detect amyloid in the brains of living people.[16] Using a chemical called PIB, named after its city of origin, they discovered that when PIB, designed to stick to amyloid, is injected into the bloodstream it lights up deposits of amyloid in the brain that can be seen by brain scanning techniques. This test became the gold standard of amyloid detection and has remained so since its discovery.

But like so many advances, it is not without drawbacks. Roughly half of senior people (age 60 and over) without any obvious signs of dementia also have significant amounts of PIB uptake in their brains. Based on these and other findings there is now an emerging view that amyloid deposits are likely to be part of the disease process but not the initial cause. The best guess right now is that amyloid may contribute to the later stages of a disease process that begins earlier, possibly even decades earlier.

The amyloid hypothesis has focused attention on the amyloid peptides that are derived from a protein of unknown function, but the tau protein is also a prominent component of impaired brains. Tau binds to and stabilizes structures called microtubules inside the axons of neurons that help maintain their shape and function. By mechanisms still unknown, tau proteins become chemically modified and create the tangles that are unable to stabilize the neuronal axons. Recently it has become possible to identify aggregates of modified tau in the brains of living people using the same brain scanning technology that was developed for the detection of amyloid. Scans of the brains of people with the early stages of dementia show that tau aggregates are indeed located in the parts the brain involved in cognition. Some believe that the tau proteins more adequately reflect brain damage than their amyloid partners.

There is much to support the idea that brain damage of dementia is related to the accumulation of amyloid and tau, but the story as we now know it is incomplete. Cognitive impairment may be caused by injuries to the brain that involve the accumulation of toxic proteins in the late stages of the disease, but there is now the realization that many undiscovered pathogenic causes may also be involved.

There are many potential toxins that damage the brain

While plaques and tangles have received the most media coverage in recent years, there are many other potentially toxic substances that the brain is exposed to. Cigarette smoking, elevated blood cholesterol levels, the consequences of diabetes mellitus, exposure to toxic metals, and even defective genes have been proposed as factors that lead to mental impairment. Mutated genes can be inherited from one's parents, but there are many examples where genes are modified by genotoxic agents [17] that we are exposed to throughout life. Ultraviolet light and other forms of radiation are thought to generate what are called reactive oxygens[18] These substances, often referred to as ROS, can modify many biological molecules including DNA molecules that create what are called somatic mutations. These mutations, created during our lifetimes, are not inherited from our parents, and it is likely that they play a significant role in the generation of chronic human diseases. How ROS affects the brain is still an open question. Some suspect that they contribute to damage that leads to the accumulation of amyloid and tau proteins.

False alarms and uncertain claims

Aluminum

People frequently ask: can I get dementia from aluminum foil? Small amounts of many metals including aluminum have been found in the brains of individuals who had a history of dementia and died of various causes. Some speculated that the metals might have contributed to the disease. Concerns have been raised regarding exposure to aluminum cooking pots, but foil, beverage cans, antacids, and antiperspirants have also been targeted. As one might imagine this issue is not without controversy, since aluminum is the most abundant metal in the human environment and has an enormous economic impact on society.

The problem became a national concern by a curious anti-aluminum campaign that began in 1913, more than a hundred years ago. Charles Truax Betts, a dentist from Ohio, unleashed a fierce campaign against the use of aluminum pots and pans that still resonates in the popular media today. Betts had a stomach problem severe enough to cause him to abandon his dental practice, and he seized on the idea that he was suffering from aluminum poisoning. He discarded all aluminum utensils in his house and within a few weeks he felt well enough to resume his practice. Convinced that aluminum was the source of his troubles, he began a decades-long campaign to alert the public to it dangers. Over time he became convinced that aluminum caused many other human illnesses including dementia. Betts self-published a booklet on the subject in 1926, but the impact of his crusade was greatly enhanced by numerous publications in *The Watchtower* a publication of the Watch Tower Bible and Tract Society of Pennsylvania that was founded in 1884. As the use of aluminum products became more prevalent the anti-aluminum crusade extended beyond kitchen-ware and included the items described above. The potential to exploit this fear was not lost on manufacturers of aluminum-free kitchen products. Even present-day advertisements continue to fuel this controversy.

The bottom line: it is highly unlikely that aluminum plays any role in the pathogenesis of human dementia. Numerous studies of aluminum-containing antacids have not found any connection with dementia. Similarly, there is no increase in the prevalence of AD in individuals with occupational exposure with aluminum, nor is there any evidence that aluminum-containing underarm antiperspirants or cosmetics increase the risk of AD. Recognizing that it is always difficult to prove a negative association with a complex human disease, a recent 2015 report of a survey of multiple studies concludes that the findings do not support an association between aluminum intake and Alzheimer's disease. [19] But a cautionary note is added: more long-term studies should still be carried out.

Mercury and Dental Fillings

Even more improbable is the suggestion that the mercury in dental fillings might be toxic to the brain. Dental amalgams have been used for more than 150 years in hundreds of millions of people around the world. Certain types of mercury are well known neurotoxins that accumulate in fish that live in polluted waters. The notorious Minamata fish problem first revealed in 1956 in Japan is a good example. The people in Minamata City in Kumamoto had been exposed to methyl mercury, a highly toxic substance in industrial wastewater that had been dumped into a nearby sea since the 1930s. Children came down with neurological diseases as did the local cat population that had eaten contaminated fish scraps. High levels of mercury were found in the hair samples of the sick people. The evidence linking some forms of mercury to neurological disease is firm and unequivocal, but dental fillings are made of an amalgam of mercury composed of mercury, silver and tin, and do not contain the toxic methyl form.

CHAPTER 3

BLOOD VESSEL DAMAGE

What has come to be known as Alzheimer's dementia dates back to the early 1900s. Was this a new disease that reflected the stresses of modern life or was it the renaming of a problem that has long plagued the human species? The answer is certainly the latter. References to dementia go back to ancient sources too numerous to list here, but in the era of modern medicine which began in 19th century Europe the prevailing view was that brain damage leading to dementia was the result of arteriosclerosis or "hardening of the arteries". This was referred to as vascular dementia. Even Alzheimer subscribed to this view in 1894, a decade before he discovered the plaques that he called amyloid. Unfortunately, the term arteriosclerosis was loosely applied to many forms of mental incapacity in the elderly, leading to the notion that it was a property of old age or a form of what was called senile dementia.

It is well known that strokes result when large blood vessels in the brain are blocked by blood clots causing what are called cerebral infarcts or sites of dead tissue that were fed by the blocked arteries. These vessels can also be damaged by arteriosclerosis. Before the deposits of amyloid were discovered, arteriosclerosis was considered the most likely cause of dementia. It was assumed that the brain was damaged the same way atherosclerotic plaques cause coronary artery disease and heart attacks.

Blocked small blood vessels may be the first step to mental impairment

George Bartzokis, a professor of psychiatry at the University of California Los Angeles pointed out that the human brain has an important advantage over the brains of non-human primates; electrical signals in the human brain travel much faster from cell to cell because their "wires" (axons) are better insulated. The axons of many critical neurons are surrounded by a layer of material called myelin that allows electrical signals to travel one hundred times faster in axons that have this insulation than those that don't. This provides great information processing ability to the human brain and explains how we can perform so many different mental functions more or less at the same time.

Bartzokis further proposed that damage to these protective myelin sheaths might account for the earliest stages of brain damage. [20] And this proved to be the case. Parts of the brain with damaged myelin are commonly found in bundles of nerves that transmit signals throughout the brain. If they are surrounded by damaged small blood vessels, the two together slow down the speed of electrical transmission through the affected circuits. This explains why many affected people speak haltingly and are often referred to as having "senior moments".

It is reasonable to ask which came first damage to the myelin sheathes of the axons or damage to the small blood vessels? Smart money would bet on blood vessel damage as the primary event since it is well known that blocking blood flow will certainly deprive brain cells of nourishment and oxygen.

The evolutionary development of the human brain gives us many advantages, but it comes with a high cost: It is extremely dependent on an adequate supply of energy in the form of nutrients and oxygen. The reason is clear: energy and oxygen are needed to generate the electricity and move it from cell to cell at such high speeds throughout the brain. The circulating blood supplies oxygen and nutrients, particularly glucose, so it is no surprise that the brain receives more blood than any other organ. It also explains why the sudden catastrophic loss of blood flow to the brain, known as a stroke, is so destructive.

What causes blood vessel damage?

The most common cause of blood vessel damage that occurs throughout the body is a process called inflammation [21]. Everyone who has had a wound or a bacterial infection has seen the tell-tale signs of inflammation. The injured site appears reddish and swollen and is warm to the touch. These signs of inflammation, recognized by the Greeks centuries ago, are what causes arthritic joints to swell and become painful. It is why lungs afflicted by pneumonia cause breathing distress. Circulating blood leukocytes collect at sites of inflammation and migrate into the damaged tissue. What they do depends on what causes the damage. If the infection is caused by bacteria, the accumulating leukocytes ingest the bacteria and clear up the wound. This activity it is beneficial to the body and is the basis for our ability to survive on this contaminated planet.

But inflammation is not always beneficial. In conditions referred to as auto-immune diseases, an unwanted inflammatory response develops that damages the body's normal tissue rather than combating alien bacteria. If this process is prolonged as it often is in many common autoimmune diseases the affected joint or organ is severely compromised. Many different forms of arthritis are caused by inflammatory reactions, and there is good reason to believe that blood vessels in the brain are also subject to such damage.

Blood vessels can also be damaged by physical trauma. Hits to the head may induce what is called traumatic encephalopathy which is accompanied by damage to the small blood vessels. Damage to both large and smaller blood vessels has also been attributed to high blood pressure. How this happens is unclear, but the incidence of strokes is significantly decreased as a result of antihypertensive medications.

HIV- associated dementia

Not generally recognized as a cause of dementia is infection by the HIV-AIDS virus [22]. Individuals who have been successfully treated by anti-retroviral therapy now have extended lifetimes; however a significant number suffer from moderate cognitive impairment even among those who have achieved viral suppression as a result of optimal therapy. Many with advanced HIV-associated dementia suffer from an inability to complete complex tasks, suffer delayed speech output, loss of initiative, and impaired fine motor skills. Some affected individuals have signs typical of Alzheimer's dementia including the presence of amyloid plaques in their brains. However, the correlation between the cognitive impairment and HIV viral loads is not high suggesting that the pathogenesis of the HIV version involves more than just neurotoxicity of the HIV virus. It is now generally recognized that HIV–related dementia is due to persistent inflammation in the brain due to immune reactions to chronic viral infection. This is an example where inflammation is clearly related to the development of cognitive impairments.

CHAPTER 4

POSSIBLE TREATMENTS

Drugs that improve brain functions

Treatments that have been pursued over the years have been based on how neuroscientists view the organization of the brain and how it functions. The current view is that the human brain is organized in what is called a distributed network in which each brain cell makes thousands of connections with other brain cells. Rather than operating as individual pathways every part of the brain is potentially connectable to every other part. And this makes sense when we consider how holistic the brain works. Our brains are also heavily electrified. Every thought we have or every image we recognize and remember depends on sparks of electricity that travel from one collection of brain cells to many others. A waking brain no matter what it is doing is a perpetual storm of electrical activity. During sleep the electrical waves are more subdued but never shut down.

As described earlier, electrical sparks that move across cell bodies travel at speeds that seem as swift as light itself, but how they pass from cell to cell is another matter. The brain is composed of many different cell types, but the ones that help us think, plan, and remember are called neurons. They have special structures that are designed to carry information from one part of the brain to another. The basic functional unit is composed of two neurons that are linked together, one that sends information and the other that receives it. Both are

21

connected together by extensions of the cell body called axons and dendrites.

A schematic of this arrangement is shown below

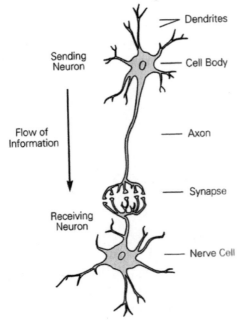

Thoughts are electric currents that travel from one neuron to another. They do this by passing down the axon so that the electric charge reaches the connecting link to the receiving neuron. The actual connection takes place through small finger-like structures that face apposing finger-like structures (called dendrites) of the receiving neuron. This connection is called a synapse, the business part of the connection. At this site the sending neuron releases chemicals called neurotransmitters [27] into the space that separates the two cells, causing the receiving dendrites to be stimulated. This is the way information is transmitted from one cell to another, a process that is repeated millions of times throughout the brain.

Scientists believe that dementia involves the loss of function of critical synapses of impaired brains. Some believe that this impairment is caused by the amyloid peptides that block the connection, while another view suggests that there may be a loss of neurotransmitter molecules that do the actual signaling, an idea that led to the first treatment for dementia.

Decades ago it was thought that mental impairments might be due to a deficiency in some of these neurotransmitter molecules. One specific one called acetylcholine was found to be reduced in certain parts of the brain that were thought to be active in memory. In the 1980s this inspired Leon Thal a neurologist at the University of California San Diego to search for ways to increase the amount of this substance in the brains of people suffering from dementia. He developed a compound called Tacrin that was designed to increase the amount of acetylcholine by blocking its breakdown. This drug was first approved by the FDA in 1993, but because of unacceptable side effects it was replaced by a compound called Aricept which is still one of the most widely prescribed drugs for dementia. Many versions of Aricept are now available, some are believed to enhance cognitive ability in the early stages of dementia, but none are able to arrest the cause of the disease. Unfortunately, the effects of Aricept and compounds like it are transient, and they do not affect the underlying disease process.

Solving the amyloid problem

Most investigators who study dementia feel that amyloid must play some role in Alzheimer's dementia, and therefore they consider it a therapeutic target even if it is not the sole cause of the disease. Why amyloid accumulates in the brains of senior citizens is a most perplexing question that until recently we couldn't answer. However, some recent experiments by investigators at Washington University in St. Louis have provided some intriguing new data. They devised ways to study amyloid in the brains of living people and discovered that large amounts of amyloid are made by the brain each day, confirming its important role in normal brain function. They also found that amyloid drains out of the brain while we sleep, an interesting observation that still remains unexplained.

Other investigators exploring this drainage process discovered that the path out of the brain that amyloid takes is along the smallest blood vessels of the brain. This is particularly interesting since these are the same vessels that when damaged block blood flow into the brain in the early stages of dementia. The question remains to be explored is whether damaged blood vessels also block the drainage of amyloid out of the brain. If so, this could explain why amyloid accumulates to levels high enough to form plaques.

Basically, we have three options to deal with amyloid accumulations:

1. We can try to find ways to block amyloid production.

2. We can try to block whatever toxic action it might have on the brain.

3. We can try to remove it from diseased brains.

Blocking amyloid production

In principle blocking amyloid production should be the easiest to achieve since we know a great deal about how the brain makes it. Amyloid is produced by highly specialized enzymes called secretases that convert larger protein molecules into smaller fragments known as peptides. Several steps are required for the secretase enzymes to generate the small amyloid peptides, and each could be blocked by a specific drug. A number of compounds have been created by pharmaceutical companies that are able to reduce amyloid to very low levels. But so far none have proved to be useful clinically. The reasons for their failure vary with the compound. Some have unacceptable side effects, others just don't work as expected. Moreover, careful studies have revealed that most patients with dementia do not suffer from amyloid over-production. Nevertheless, this approach is still being pursued in the hope that compounds can be found that reduce amyloid levels and still have tolerable side effects.

Blocking toxic actions

Option number two, blocking the toxic action of amyloid has also not been successful. Here we have a different problem. Despite more than two decades of laboratory research we still do not know precisely how amyloid damages brain cells. Without knowing this there is no obvious way to block its toxicity. Great excitement was generated more than two decades ago when it was discovered that human amyloid could be produced in the brains of experimental animals. Traditionally animal models of disease have led the way to the study of human disease and in many cases, they have allowed scientists to systematically study the course of a disease process from its beginning and in doing so were able to study ways to interrupt its progression. These animal models have also proved useful as ways to test potential therapies. Unfortunately, studies of amyloid in experimental animals have produced confusing results, and many investigators question whether their findings are relevant to the human problem. At present there are no FDA approved drugs that can block the toxic actions of amyloid in human patients.

Immunity as Treatment: A Multi-billion dollar Gamble

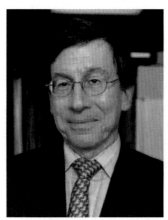

**Dale Schenk
(1957-2016)**

The third option, removing amyloid from diseased brains, is now being aggressively pursued because of an unexpected experimental result obtained more than two decades ago. In the late 1990s Dale Schenk chief scientific officer at Elan Corporation and his collaborators reported a scientific discovery that raised the eyebrows of the entire Alzheimer's research community. Their findings suggested that amyloid deposits in the brains of experimental animals could be removed by immune therapy [28].

The idea of using our immune system to combat disease has a long history. In the late 1700s the disease we know as smallpox was a major killer of young people and was as greatly feared as Alzheimer's dementia is today. Edward Jenner, an English country doctor, saw that cattle farmers were not dying from small pox during the epidemic of 1788. He also realized that cattle suffered from a disease related to smallpox, called cowpox, but it was much less virulent. Jenner also noticed that young women who milked cows infected with cowpox had far fewer smallpox scars than women who were not exposed to sick cows. Jenner guessed, correctly as it turned out, that fluid extracted from cowpox sores protected against human smallpox. Since the first anti-smallpox treatment was derived from cows (vacca) it was called a vaccine. Since then any preparation used as a preventive inoculation to confer immunity against a specific disease is referred to as a vaccine.

Our understanding of vaccination has come a long way since Jenner's time, witness the highly effective polio vaccines and most recently the Ebola vaccine. But in every case of an infectious disease there was a specific biologic target (often a virus) that could be used to create the vaccine. Dale Schenk and his collaborators decided to repeat the Jenner experiment on laboratory animals using amyloid as the test material in the hopes of generating antibodies that would clear amyloid out of their brains. Positive results from these animal studies encouraged Schenk to carry out a pilot clinical study on a small number of patients, a trial that turned out to be both a success and a failure. Some of the patients who were vaccinated did develop antibodies to the amyloid material, and after they died, from other causes, autopsy studies revealed that amyloid deposits in some of the treated brains were depleted. Unfortunately, vaccination was found to provoke an immune reaction in the form of encephalitis in some of the patients, so this clinical trial was immediately ended. But the idea that immune therapy might be effective if it could be made safe convinced Schenk and his colleagues to persevere. They decided to immunize normal animals with amyloid and use the antibodies harvested from these animals to treat other diseased animals. They obtained remarkable results: the added antibodies removed most of the amyloid from the brains of the treated animals.

Using antibodies to treat chronic human diseases has a long history in clinical medicine. Rheumatoid arthritis, a chronic disease that affects the small joints in the hands and feet, has been treated with a number of different antibodies, each directed against a specific cause of the disease. Success of these treatments depends on the ability of the antibodies to neutralize the toxic factors that cause the problem. This approach offers a way to remove amyloid from the brains of living people, and, hopefully, will be a way to rescue damaged brain cells.

A staggering amount of money has been devoted to the development of antibodies that might be able to remove amyloid from the brains of living patients. After many years of clinical trials it has been shown that antibodies can remove amyloid from the brains of affected people. But whether this approach can restore mental impairments is yet to be determined. Clinical trials continue to be pursued despite many disappointing failures.

CHAPTER 5

PREVENTION IS THE MOST REALISTIC NEAR TERM GOAL

How can we blunt this impending catastrophe? Based on what we now know we can predict that at least a third (and maybe more) of elderly people at risk to develop dementia will benefit from the preventive measures that are outlined below. Based on this estimate we might be able to rescue millions of people who would otherwise develop mental impairments.

In order to achieve this goal, we have to address three issues:

1. We must try to identify the most likely causes that lead to mental impairment. There are many more potential causes of brain damage than simply the overabundance of toxic amyloid. Having some idea of possible causes will help us design preventive strategies.

2. We have to learn which lifestyles are most likely to maintain our cognitive capacities. There is no doubt that the way we live our lives matters a great deal in the likelihood of our developing serious mental impairments in our later years. What we eat, what medications we take, and how active we are, both physically and mentally, all matter.

3. Perhaps most important of all for elderly populations, we have to learn how to rejuvenate the brains of aging people. There is no doubt

that even healthy brains start to run downhill even in the absence of disease. Neuroscientists have discovered that adult brains can be changed for the better provided that appropriate measures are followed.

Dealing with toxic proteins and unknown causes

The major pharmaceutical companies have focused on removal of toxic proteins from damaged brains, both as a therapeutic approach and a preventive measure. Billions of dollars have been spent on the development of antibodies that are designed to remove amyloid in living patients who are at the different stages of the disease. So far success has been limited. These efforts face a conundrum: lack of success can be explained in a number of ways. It is possible even likely that the treatments were administered too late in the course of the disease. Some even propose that patients who show evidence of amyloid in their brains are already too far along in the disease to be rescued. This implies that treatment should begin in people without any symptoms. This means that cognitively normal people may have to undergo treatments for many years, a daunting prospect. Other critics contend that amyloid is not the prime cause of disease. The presence of amyloid deposits seen in the brains of normal people convinces many that these deposits are either benign or are the result of other changes in the brain that cause their accumulation.

But toxic proteins are not the only possible cause of brain damage. Toxic substances in the environment called free radicals that have the capacity to damage DNA are widely regarded as a major cause of many chronic diseases. For many people cigarette smoking adds to this problem. The consequences of diabetes mellitus, high lipid levels and cholesterol, and high blood pressure all have the capacity to contribute to brain damage to varying degrees. We also have to consider the exposure to heavy metals such as mercury, lead, and possibly even aluminum as contributing factors, although as described earlier there is little evidence that our exposure to aluminum contributes to dementia. The point of listing all these possibilities is to convince the reader that Alzheimer's dementia and related diseases have many possible causes, some often seemingly inconsequential, but they can contribute to more serious problems when they are incremental. This makes it unlikely that any one single treatment will be effective and explains why so many clinical trials have variable outcomes.

Blocking blood vessel damage

As described earlier, inflammation damages small blood vessels throughout the body including the brain. There are many known anti-inflammatory agents that could be used to reduce inflammation in the brain. Several specific anti-inflammatory agents have been tested, but there were no obvious differences between a specific agent and a placebo control. However, as emphasized earlier, single agents may not be effective for many reasons. Unfortunately, the intense anti-amyloid focus has attracted so much attention in recent years that few investigators have explored ways to block inflammatory reactions in the small blood vessels of the brain that are known to be damaged during the early stages of the disease. This is an area of investigation that deserves much more attention.

Blood vessels can also be damaged by trauma, an issue that is now being pursued in studies of traumatic encephalopathy of professional athletes and those who are exposed to explosive warfare. Since these studies involve severe repetitive injuries they don't address how less traumatic injury can damage blood vessels in critical parts of the brain. Damaged blood vessels might also affect the ability of the brain to drain amyloid deposits out of the brain as described earlier.

Uncontrolled high blood pressure has long been considered a source of cardiovascular injury throughout the body, and there is no reason why this condition might not also affect blood vessels of the brain. But clinical trials to address this question have produced conflicting results with regard to dementia. Some investigators found elevated blood pressure to be a contributing factor in the development of dementia, but other studies failed to support this. However recent studies have confirmed that elevated blood pressure might be a contributing factor to brain injury if high blood pressure levels occur while affected people are in their middle ages between 35 and 50 years old. [29] Older people with the same degree of high blood pressure seem not to have the same serious consequences.

Lifestyle modifications as preventive measures

How we live has a lot to do with how our brain will function in later life. There is no doubt that what we eat, what medications we take, and how active we are both mentally and physically matter a great deal. We could devote a whole book discussing all the ways that diets and medications are thought to influence how our brain changes in later life, yet a relatively brief summary would more than adequately cover what we actually know.

The Mediterranean diet

The Mediterranean diet, widely acclaimed by many, involves the consumption of fruit, vegetables, legumes, and olive oil along with moderate consumptions of dairy products. Meat (especially red meat) consumption is strongly discouraged. Its name is derived from the dietary practices followed by people living along the shores of the Mediterranean Sea, these include Greece, France, Spain, and Italy as well as parts of North Africa. Since it includes the practices of many different cultures there is no unified consensus as to what the Mediterranean diet actually is, but the main components are the same across all the countries.

Ancel Keys a scientist at the University of Minnesota spent time in Italy during World War II. At that time he noticed the large numbers of centenarians who lived in the small towns of southern Italy. During later studies he discovered that the relatively poor citizens of these towns seem to be healthier than their own relatives who immigrated to the United States decades earlier. Suspecting that the difference was due to the diets of the two different populations, Keys initiated studies of populations of several other countries and concluded that the diets of people living in the Mediterranean regions accounted for the much lower incidence of cardiovascular disease. He and others discovered that people with lower levels of coronary artery disease also had low levels of cholesterol in their blood. This was attributed to their diets of olive oil, pasta, vegetables, garlic and very low amounts of meat. This became known as the Mediterranean diet.

Keys' focus was on the role of nutrition in cardiovascular disease, including coronary artery disease and heart attacks, but we now realize that the same dietary considerations apply equally well to normal cognition and impaired cognition that lead to dementia. More recent studies of nutrition and dementia have led to proposals for three different but related diets, these are known as the Mediterranean diet (MeDi), the DASH diet (dietary approaches to stop hypertension), and most recently the MIND diet (Mediterranean –DASH diet) as possible interventions for neurodegenerative disease.)

The DASH diet focused on the reduction of salt and other practices that contribute to high blood pressure, while, the MIND diet seeks to combine the best of both and includes green leafy vegetables, nuts, beans, whole grains, fish, poultry, olive oil, and wine. In addition to proposing what one should eat a number of interdictions have also been proposed. These include eliminating sugary drinks, refined carbohydrates, foods rich in high trans fats, and otherwise highly processed foods.

The Mediterranean diet has been characterized as a lifestyle rather than simply a diet since it includes people eating together in a social event that brings together family and friends and involves people who are physically active. The prevailing view is that the Mediterranean diet lowers the risk of cognitive decline by reducing the risk of developing cardiovascular disease. The Mediterranean diet is not considered a low-fat diet. The fat content ranges from 28–40% of the total dietary intake, but it is low in saturated fatty acids due to its low content of animal meats and processed foods. Olive oil (oleic acid), a beneficial monounsaturated fatty acid, is the major contributor to this fat content which makes it a healthy diet regardless of its high fat content.

While these attributes support the widely held belief that prudent diets are good for both the body and the mind, it is important to ask whether critical studies have been done to confirm these notions. Unfortunately, studies of people who follow this diet in non-Mediterranean countries such as the United States report mixed results. Contrary to the findings of people who actually live in the Mediterranean region where randomized clinical trials do show positive changes, some studies of Americans who follow this practice do show protective effect, but other studies do not. The prevailing view that Mediterranean diets lower the risk of cardiovascular disease is partly due to the high content of B vitamins, folic acid, and omega-3 fatty acids, all of which contribute an anti-inflammatory and anti-oxidative function.

Vitamins and dementia

Vitamins are naturally occurring substances that are present in foods in extremely small amounts that are needed for many different biological functions. A characteristic feature of many of the vitamins is that their absence from the diet can cause specific deficiencies some of which cause serious problems. Historically seamen on long-distance voyages in the 1700s suffered from a variety of problems due to defective blood vessels, known as scurvy, which physicians in the British navy realized might be prevented by the intake of limes. In the 1930s this protective effect was found to be due to ascorbic acid, now known as vitamin C, a substance necessary for the synthesis of the protein called collagen that provides structure for blood vessels, bones, and ligaments.

The introduction of vitamin C in various forms completely eliminated scurvy, and since then many have considered it a protective substance that might have other applications. A notorious example was the claim by a highly regarded scientist named Linus Pauling, twice a Nobel Prize winner, who proposed that vitamin C could cure the common cold. Nothing could be more welcome to those who suffer this irritating but not life-threatening problem, and millions of people took to ingesting large quantities of vitamin C, hoping to either prevent or reduce the complications. Many carefully designed clinical trials showed unequivocally that the ingestion of large amounts of vitamin C did not prevent the development of viral-induced upper respiratory infections or the so-called common cold. Regardless, and uncharacteristically of a great scientist, Pauling refused to accept the results of these studies. It is not clear whether his ideas influenced the general public, but to this day vast numbers of people use inappropriate amounts of vitamin C to prevent colds and many other ailments. Fortunately, ingesting moderate amounts of vitamin C is not a problem for most people, but excessive amounts can cause serious complications including kidney stones. Vitamin C is probably the most popular single vitamin supplement, yet it is present in plentiful amounts in many fruits and vegetables. Many nutritionists question the routine use of vitamin C for people who have reasonable food intakes.

Beriberi is another disease of nutritional deficiency, more prevalent in the past than now, that signals the importance of thiamine, now known as vitamin B1. Because thiamine has so many different roles in the body's metabolism and in the functioning of the nervous system, lacking it can cause many symptoms including swelling of the lower limbs, various neurological deficits, and in some cases heart failure. There are many B vitamins and all of them can be supplied by a well-balanced diet.

Vitamin D is an important exception. Unlike most of the other vitamins, vitamin D is not present in most foods. It is found in cod liver oil, fish, mushrooms, and eggs, but the quantities are small except in the case of cod liver oil. Our bodies need vitamin D to absorb calcium which is necessary to promote bone growth. Total vitamin deficiency results in soft bones in children (rickets) and fragile misshapen bones in adults (osteomalacia).

A substantial amount of vitamin D is made in the skin due to exposure to the sun, but it has been estimated that a significant fraction of the United States population is vitamin D deficient. This condition is likely to be worse among people with darker skin living in northern zones as pigment screens out the protective effects of the sun. Vitamin D deficiency is basically a disease of neglect since it depends upon people either not getting enough sun exposure or an appropriate supplement. A daily intake of 1000 IU of cholecalciferol (D3) may be needed for most adults, particularly postmenopausal women and older men.

Vitamin E is more controversial. This vitamin is thought to have a role in preventing cardiovascular disease by inhibiting the oxidation of low-density lipoprotein (LDL). Several epidemiologic studies have indicated that high dietary intake of vitamin E is associated with high serum concentrations of alpha tocopherol and lower rates of ischemic heart disease. Because vitamin E is known to have antioxidant activity it is assumed that it acts on many different pathogenic processes. However, unlike vitamin D, there is abundant amounts of vitamin E in most common foods, for most people supplements of vitamin E are should be taken with caution.

The Multi-Vitamin Problem

Half of all American adults—including 70 percent of those age 65 and older—take a multivitamin or another vitamin or mineral supplement regularly. The total price tag exceeds $12 billion per year, money that many nutrition experts say might be better spent on nutrient-packed foods like fruit, vegetables, whole grains, and low-fat dairy products.

- In an editorial in the journal Annals of Internal Medicine titled "Enough Is Enough: Stop Wasting Money on Vitamin and Mineral Supplements," researchers reviewed evidence about supplements, including three very recent studies. [30] An analysis of research involving 450,000 people, found that multivitamins did not reduce risk for heart disease or cancer.

- A study that tracked the mental functioning and multivitamin use of 5,947 men for 12 years found that multivitamins did not reduce risk for mental declines such as memory loss or slowed-down thinking.

- A study of 1,708 heart attack survivors who took a high-dose multivitamin or placebo for up to 55 months showed that rates of later heart attacks, heart surgeries and deaths were similar in the two groups.

Antioxidants

Antioxidants are widely regarded as potential protective factors largely because they can neutralize the damage caused by reactive oxygens described earlier. The most commonly used antioxidants are vitamins A, C, and E. They are found in many fruits, vegetables, and berries, or they can be taken as supplements. People who reported a greater intake of fruits and vegetables were found to have a lower risk of cardiovascular disease and better cognitive function. It was also found that the protective effect of vitamin E was strongest when individuals consume vitamin E from dietary sources rather than from dietary supplements. The suggestion here is that consuming fruits and vegetables was a more effective way of ingesting active vitamins than the synthetic forms.

Many other natural substances have anti-oxidative activity. Compounds called flavonoids that are found in red wine and berries have been associated with reduced rates of cognitive decline. But, as was true in the case of the other putative protective substances, several studies have suggested that progression of mild cognitive impairment to more severe forms was not significantly impacted by vitamin E treatment.

Cognitive enhancers: Do they work for dementia

Caffeine is the most widely consumed psychoactive drug in the world. It is estimated that 85% of American adults consume some form of caffeine daily in the form of coffee, tea, and cola. Milk chocolate made from cocoa beans has a small amount of caffeine, but dark chocolate has 2 to 3 times the amount of caffeine as coffee.[31] At normal doses caffeine generally improves reaction time, awareness, concentration, and motor coordination. The amount of caffeine needed to produce these effects varies from person to person. Since the desired effects of a moderate dose can last three or four hours, it is difficult to determine whether it enhances learning and memory. Whether caffeine has a positive effect on dementia is considered possible by some, but the evidence is inconclusive.[32]

Resveratrol is a complex plant product found in the skin of grapes, blueberries, and raspberries that is believed to have anti-oxidant activity. Research interest in the therapeutic relevance of resveratrol and its popular appeal originated from its association with the "French Paradox" in the early 1990s.[33] It has been claimed that the consumption of red wine on a regular basis may be related to a lower risk of developing dementia.

Interest in resveratrol got a big boost when it was reported that some formulations of resveratrol acted on an enzyme that was involved in aging. This prompted the formation of a biotechnology company called Sirtris Pharmaceuticals based in Cambridge Massachusetts to develop specific anti-aging formulations. After other investigators carried out similar studies, doubts were raised as to whether their products had the desired effects. A review of existing resveratrol research in 2016 [33] demonstrated there was not enough evidence to demonstrate its effect on longevity nor could there be recommendations for intake beyond the amount normally obtained through dietary sources, estimated as being less than 4 mg/day. Most of the research showing positive effects has been done on animals, with insufficient clinical research on humans. It was also noted that its alleged protective effects on heart disease, cancer, and cognition have not been confirmed.

Curcumin is a polyphenolic compound obtained from turmeric, the spice that gives curry its yellow color. It has been used in India for thousands of years as a food flavoring and preservative and as a herbal remedy to treat a variety of human illnesses, presumably due to its ability to block inflammation or reduce oxidative stress. It has also been claimed that curcumin decreases amyloid production and possibly even neutralizes its toxic activities. Turmeric has been reputed to possess neuroprotective effects, and some epidemiological studies support a link between dietary curry consumption and improved cognitive performance in elderly populations.

Despite a long tradition of many different medical uses, carefully controlled clinical studies have failed to show the efficacy of curcumin as either a protective component or treatment for an ongoing illness. According to a 2017 review of over 120 studies [34], curcumin has not been successful in any clinical trial, leading the authors to conclude that "curcumin is an unstable, reactive, compound and, therefore, a highly improbable therapy".

The results of an epidemiological study comparing the low incidence of dementia in a rural community in India to subjects in rural Pennsylvania is often cited as evidence that a diet containing turmeric is beneficial. However, even the authors of the oft-cited study cautioned against over-interpretation of their results given the relatively short duration of the study, the small number of incident cases, and other confounding factors.

Despite this abundant negative evidence, massive numbers of scientific manuscripts are still published regularly, testimony to the powers of commercialization and abetted by the hope of many people that ancient natural products have special powers not easily recognized by modern science.

Ginkgo Biloba

Ginkgo biloba has been used in traditional Chinese medicine for thousands of years, and today it is one of the most popular herbal supplements. Ginkgo biloba extract is collected from the dried leaves of the plant and is used for a variety of ailments. Gingko contains high levels of the antioxidant flavonoids and terpenoids that are believed to provide protection against oxidative cell damage from harmful free radicals. Its advocates believe that ginkgo improves cognitive function because it promotes good blood circulation in the brain and protects the brain from neuronal damage. Like most herbal products, nobody knows exactly how ginkgo biloba works.

Some studies show a marked reduction in the rate of cognitive decline in people with dementia using ginkgo, but others fail to replicate this finding. A large review of research concluded that supplementing with ginkgo did not result in any measurable improvements in memory, executive function or attention capacity.[35]

Herbal remedies such as curcumin and ginkgo biloba are difficult to evaluate for many reasons. They are usually composed of many different substances, most inadequately characterized, and because they are herbal products and considered as dietary supplements they do not have to be evaluated and approved by the Food and Drug Administration (FDA) to ensure that they are safe and effective. A recent summary points out the problems we face trying to evaluate the vast number of herbal extracts. [36]

"Botanical dietary supplements (BDS) are complex mixtures of phytochemicals exhibiting complex pharmacology and posing complex research challenges. For 25 years, clinical pharmacologists researching BDS have confronted a litany of issues unlike those encountered with conventional medications. Foundational to these concerns is the Dietary Supplement Health and Education Act of 1994, which exempted BDS from premarket safety and efficacy trials. In the ensuing period, safety concerns regarding multi-ingredient products formulated as "proprietary blends" and herb-drug interactions have garnered significant attention and idiosyncrasies unique to individual compounds. Despite a quarter century of public use, healthcare professionals still know little about such dietary supplements, thus it falls to industry, government, and academia to join forces in promoting a new paradigm for research and product development."

Physical activity: How important is it for a healthy brain?

It is generally recognized that physical activity has many benefits for older people. It has obvious benefits on the body itself, active muscles grow and provide increased mobility and muscular strength, and moderately vigorous activity greatly increases one's sense of fitness. It is widely assumed that the beneficial effects of vigorous exercise largely depend upon improvements in the cardiovascular system, but this assumption is open to question, since many studies demonstrate that aerobic fitness training enhances the capacities of the brain itself independent of cardiovascular fitness.

How this works is still unclear, but there are several ways in which moderately vigorous physical activity can help the brain function. Increasing blood flow to the brain provides more oxygen and glucose for its normal functions. Factors that protect the brain are activated during exercise and promote nerve cell growth that lead to more effective synaptic connections. There is also evidence that certain chemicals that activate the brain such as dopamine, norepinephrine, and even lactate contribute to improving memory functions.

The type of exercise matters, as well as its intensity, duration, and frequency. The term aerobic exercise is widely used to describe activities that require oxygen, even though all activities require oxygen, some do more than others. Examples of aerobic exercises include running, jogging, swimming, cycling, and even walking. Aerobic exercises are performed at a moderate level of intensity over a relatively long time. For example, running a long distance at a moderate pace is an aerobic exercise, but sprinting is not.

Activities that are not considered aerobic involve muscles acting against resistance or involve weight-bearing activities. Muscles that contract against strong resistance promote the secretion of chemicals called myokines [37] that act on the muscles in a variety of ways. Some increase the growth of muscle tissue, some activate different metabolic processes, and some are thought to exert anti-inflammatory functions. The amount of myokines that are secreted depends upon the amount of muscle that is contracted and the duration and intensity of the contractions.

How Exercise grows the Brain

A recent Science Times section of the New York Times[38] proposed a novel suggestion: "Want to be 30 years younger (biologically speaking)? Try decades of exercise". This article describes a recent study published in the Journal of Applied Physiology that reports the effects of lifelong aerobic exercises on a select set of senior septuagenarians who had had carefully documented histories of active aerobic exercise over 50+ years. These active seniors were found to have much higher aerobic capacities than most people their age, and in terms of fitness their muscles were described as matching those of 25-year-olds. Another interesting finding was the discovery that their muscles contained many more small blood vessels than are usually found in people in their age group. This meant that their individual muscle cells were receiving more oxygen and nutrients then less vascularized tissue. Since the growth of blood vessels requires specific factors, (the three most significant are vascular endothelial growth factor (VEGF), brain-derived neurotrophic factor (BDNF), and nerve growth factor (NGF). These investigators suggested that vigorous exercise promoted higher growth factor levels than expected at their ages. And this turned out to be the case when appropriate studies were done.

Why is this relevant to exercise and dementia?

The idea that the aging brain can lose its blood supply is an old one. In the early 1900s it was proposed that a decrease in blood supply to the brain contributed to the pathogenesis of dementia. It was called vascular dementia. In support of this idea was the observation that some elderly individuals had greatly reduced numbers of blood capillaries in different parts of their brains. Later it was found that the brains of some Alzheimer's patients also had reduced numbers of capillaries, but it was difficult to determine whether their loss represents a consequence of other disease processes.

These decades-old observations have recently been supported by some provocative experimental studies on aging animals. Scientists in Japan discovered that rats developed significant muscle loss as they age, a process called sarcopenia. Careful study of the blood vessels of their leg muscles show a remarkable change in the number blood capillaries when compared with younger animals. Blood vessels that supply the nerves to the aging muscles were significantly diminished in number and in size.

To extend these interesting studies another set of aging rats were run on a treadmill for one hour a day for two weeks to see whether exercise would rescue the aging muscles. The results were equally dramatic. A great increase in the number of blood vessels developed after a two-week training period. Equally informative was the discovery that two critical growth factors, BDNF and VEGF, were elevated in the exercised animals, but were not detected in the sedentary ones. What we know today suggests that physical activity does indeed affect cognitive performance, but the types, duration, and intensity of the activity have yet to be determined. This explains why many studies on the effect of exercise report conflicting results.

Will thinking while exercising help?

An interesting new idea has recently been proposed: What about activating the brain while performing physical exercises? Several studies have suggested that if physical activities and mental exercises are combined, either simultaneously or sequentially, better results in cognitive performance are obtained than after either type of single training alone. The best results are obtained when the physical training involves increasing levels of difficulty. The suggestion here is that challenging physical activities will be effective if they are carried out under cognitively demanding conditions. In other words, physical activity that is considered good for the brain is most effective if it is coupled with challenges to the brain itself..

To summarize:

• Physical exercise can significantly improve cognitive function in senior adults, 50 years and older, regardless of their mental status.

• Positive benefits to cognition were achieved when exercise interventions either aerobic training or resistance exercises were combined with cognitively demanding exercises.

• The intensity and duration of physical exercises are equally important; Most improvements were obtained when physical exercises had a minimum duration of 45 minutes at moderate to vigorous intensity.

CHAPTER 6

PROBLEMS OF BEHAVIOR: PHYSICAL AND MENTAL INACTIVITY

While abnormal protein deposits and damage to small blood vessels are certainly features of brains afflicted with dementia, it is now clear that activities within the brain itself may contribute to the problem. All human brains regardless of age or sex are capable of undergoing both physical and functional changes throughout one's lifetime. This property, which neuroscientists called plasticity, reflects the ability of the brain to respond to both activity and inactivity.[23] Like muscles, which grow larger when challenged by increasing physical activity, so does the brain respond. And, like inactive muscles, inactive brains also lose their capacities if not challenged. This loss of activity is most noticeably evident in the parts of the brain that involve memory and other cognitive functions. It is estimated that fully one third of individuals with decreased cognitive capacities have issues that may be caused by disuse of these functions during one's lifetime. These changes may explain why highly educated people have lower incidence of dementia than those with lesser schooling. People who have mentally challenging occupations also have a lower incidence.

Education matters

In 1996 a group of scientists at the University of Kentucky reported a surprising finding: education and intellectual development

42

during early life was a strong predictor of cognitive function and Alzheimer's disease in old age. [24] They drew this surprising conclusion from a study of nuns who were members of the School Sisters of Notre Dame, a Catholic order in the Midwest. They reasoned that studying people who lived for many years under rigorously controlled situations with common diet, occupation, habits, and smoking history would be revealing.

Six hundred and seventy-eight nuns all approximately seventy-five years old and all free of any signs of dementia agreed to be tested every year and have their brains examined at autopsy when they died. On looking into their backgrounds, it was discovered that many of the women had hand-written autobiographies stored in church archives that were written when the women were in their early 20s, or roughly fifty years before the study began. To assess the mental state of these women at the time they wrote these pieces, the last ten sentences of each autobiography were analyzed for what the investigators called the linguistic complexity or idea content of each one. Based on this analysis, two groups of women were identified, those with high idea content, two-thirds of the total, and those with lower content, the remaining third of the group. Keep in mind that the nuns in the study whose autobiographies were analyzed were seventy-five years old and all mentally intact when the study began. Within a decade a number developed dementia and when they died autopsy studies revealed that many had AD-related pathology in their brains. This was not surprising since they were all in their late 80s or early 90s. What was unexpected however, all who developed the disease were in the lowest idea content group. These findings have since been confirmed by many other studies. Levels of education matter in terms of who gets dementia in later life. The higher the level of education one achieves the lower the incidence of dementia. One has to wonder whether this explains the connection between lesser linguistic ability of the nuns and dementia in later life.

No discussion of the nun study would be complete without recounting the life and career of Sister Mary as David Snowdon described it in a 1997 article. [25] She provided another surprise. Born in 1892 in Philadelphia to a working-class Catholic family, the first of ten children, she was forced to leave school after the eighth grade when her mother died during the birth of her tenth child. As a member of the School Sisters of Notre Dame in Baltimore, Maryland, Sister Mary taught seventh and eighth grades in public schools while at the same time earning a high school diploma at age 41. Her high school transcript indicated that she maintained an A average with a 100 in algebra and 80 in drawing. She taught school full time until she was 77 years old and then worked part time as a math teacher until she finally retired at 84. During her "retirement" she continued to follow community and world events and is described as having held court in the convent delivering lessons with grace. She became a member of the nun study and was tested regularly and was found to be cognitively intact at age 101. After her death, eight months after being tested, an autopsy of her brain revealed another surprising finding: it had all the plaques and tangles one finds in the brains of people with Alzheimer's disease. Sister Mary had no inkling of what was going on in her brain and suffered no impairment, nor were the standard brain tests at all revealing.

Paradoxes: A personal experience

Sally Lockwood Marchesi, my wife and the inspiration behind this book, was a Phi Beta Kappa graduate of Smith College who entered the Yale Medical School in 1957 as one of five women in a class of eighty. She did graduate work at Oxford University where she studied the metabolism of Vitamin B^{12} before returning to Yale for her MD degree in 1963. She then spent the next four years first at Barnes Hospital in St. Louis and then at Montefiore Hospital in New York City. This was followed by a fellowship at the National Institutes of Health in Bethesda, Md, where she did ground breaking work on the blood protein involved in hemophilia. In 1972, she returned to Yale and spent the rest of her career focusing on clinical hematology and clinical medicine, her first and greatest passion. By all accounts she was both a critical thinker and a compassionate physician.

Sometime in the 1980s Sally started burning coffee pots. Not one or two, but many. She'd turn them on and then go off to do something else. Over the years this progressed to more obvious problems which we both tried to ignore. After all she was a full time Yale professor and a mother of six children. She had lots of reasons for being forgetful.

Just as the medically trained are among the last to recognize their own health problems, just the opposite happens when they do have a problem. Often the worst possible alternatives are imagined, as Sally did, when she cried in bed on many mornings. In her mind, as well as mine, the specter of dementia was all consuming. And doctors were not at all helpful. Just as ignorant of the disease and its consequences at that time as we were, they subjected her to a barrage of tests that turned up nothing. We consulted a neurologist who had little first-hand experience with Alzheimer's disease and several psychiatrists who could only test her but offered no solutions, including one who pronounced her condition as hopeless. Back then the tools now available to diagnose dementia had not yet been invented, so it was deemed necessary to rule out every known type of dementia that might be treatable, such as vitamin B^{12} deficiency, thyroid insufficiency, and even HIV AIDS. Sally hated these tests. She was found to be anemic, and her doctors insisted that a source of bleeding be looked for, which meant she had to have a colonoscopy to rule out a gastrointestinal malignancy. Nothing was found. All these negative findings made Alzheimer's dementia the diagnosis by exclusion. Sally decided she probably had a stroke. This comforted us both since in our minds strokes were onetime events that in her case appeared to be limited. A stroke did make sense since both her uncle and father died of cardiovascular disease (her uncle at age 35 and her father at 59) so a vascular problem was a real possibility.

By the year 2000, Sally, age 64, was clinically sick and had been through a number of setbacks, both professionally and personally, that ended her career as a physician/professor. I remember the night she came home after her last teaching assignment. As she described it to me that evening, she was giving a lecture in an auditorium at the medical school using Power Point slides. Midway through her talk, when the next frame appeared on the screen, she didn't know what to say. She stood at the podium staring at the screen, probably for several minutes. She noticed the students whispering to each other, and then, one by one they left leaving her standing alone in the empty auditorium.

Sally stayed home with me for two more years, and we had our good moments. Realizing that she was unable to prepare meals on her own she relished the chance to peel potatoes or devein shrimp and insisted on washing the dishes while the meal was still in progress. She never lost her desire to matter. I soon realized that I had to monitor her showers to prevent her from turning up the hot water. She seemed to like having me help her dress. Tying her running shoes was also playful.

I quickly tied one shoe while she miss-tied the other. I then rushed to redo that before she could undo mine, while we both laughed. Near the end Sally was home with me most of the day and all of the night, yet we were both alone. She was friendly, agreeable, eager to please, but distant. To me she was already gone. I was devastated by Sally's problem. Like every other caregiver I felt completely powerless.

Education and intelligence (usually) matter

There is now convincing evidence that education and intelligence play an important role in preventing the development of dementia. Nuns who had less linguistic capacities when they were young were more likely to develop dementia 60 years later. This inverse association of mental capacity and late stage dementia also extends to levels of education and is consistent with the idea that mental capacities and the intellectual activities they support are able to counteract the gradual loss of cognitive ability that is a consequence of natural aging.

So how do we account for all the people we know who are highly intelligent yet suffer from dementia? Sally Marchesi, highly educated, with three advanced degrees, was one obvious example. Her healthy lifestyle and demanding professional activities should have been

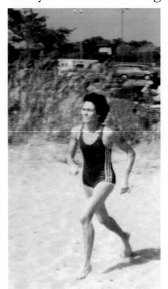

protective. Sally was a lifelong long-distance runner who was fastidious about her diet, a non-smoker who pursued many intellectual activities until she was in the late stages of her disease. In short, she had all the attributes that one would predict for a cognitively healthy person.

However, Sister Mary presented another paradox in that her 101-year-old brain contained significant amounts of amyloid plaques and tangles, yet she was totally intact mentally by all objective measurements. There are now many examples of senior people who have deposits of amyloid in their brains yet appear cognitively intact. This raises an important question: Do deposits of

Sally Lockwood Marchesi, during her adult years

amyloid alone cause dementia, or could they be a consequence of damage caused by other factors?

Cholesterol and heart disease

In many ways the link between amyloid and dementia can be compared with the association between high cholesterol levels and cardiovascular disease. Like amyloid in brains of people with dementia, deposits of cholesterol accumulate in our large arteries and are the most important cause of coronary artery disease and heart attacks. More than three decades ago studies of people with early coronary artery disease indicated that abnormal genes promoted the accumulation of cholesterol in their vessels, a discovery that placed cholesterol levels as the number one cause of coronary artery disease

However, recent new findings support an important revision of this idea. While not discounting the influence of cholesterol as a cause of damage to blood vessel walls, it is now clear that cholesterol accumulations occur after inflammatory cells invade the blood vessel walls. This places inflammation as the primary cause of atherosclerosis [26] with cholesterol an important contributing factor.

There are revealing parallels between the effects of cholesterol on coronary arteries of the heart and amyloid on the brain. Both accumulate in damaged blood vessels. This could explain why the same factors that promote cardiovascular damage also lead to dementia. The underlying cause of both conditions could be low levels of inflammation that take a long time to develop into clinically evident disease.

We don't know why the many protective factors of Sally Marchesi's life style failed to arrest the progression of her disease, nor can we explain why Sister Mary suffered no obvious consequences of her amyloid burden. Mental impairment can come about by two distinct mechanisms, one involves brain tissue damage that has irreversible consequences and the other a reduced capacity of an otherwise normal brain to function normally. Diseases that involve tissue damage impair the brain to the point of dementia and involve changes that override the effects of protective measures, regardless of their magnitude. Based on this reasoning, Sister Mary suffered no impairment even with a significant amyloid burden because it did not damage the brain irreversibly. Whatever impairments she might have suffered were compensated for by protective factors. We can only guess but they surely included vigorous intellectual activity. Because of her father's medical history, Sally Marchesi's impairment could have been due to blood vessel damage of unknown causes which could not be rescued by the same protective mechanisms. The many causes of injury to the brain described earlier explain why so many smart and physically active people become impaired despite a healthy life style.

It is possible that the single most important cause of Alzheimer's dementia will be identified, but this is an unlikely prospect. It is now clear that many pathogenic factors contribute to the development of mental impairments. Identifying any one of them would represent an important advance but dealing with any one alone without dealing with other contributing causes would not solve the problem. Indeed, as things stand right now (2019), we are at an impasse.

CHAPTER 7

QUESTIONS

Can we rejuvenate the brains of aging people?

Given the horrific predictions of mental incapacity that are predicted to affect all populations worldwide as they age, we have to ask: In the absence of effective treatments, what can be done to prevent the onset of dementia or reduce the rate of its progression? While not knowing causes is certainly a handicap for developing a treatment, it shouldn't prevent us from exploring ways to prevent the problem, particularly since we now realize that the earliest stages of cognitive impairment begin decades before symptoms are apparent and before irreversible damage has taken place. Since problems of mental incapacity are an overwhelming problem of aging people, we can start by asking why doesn't everyone over the age of 65 get the disease? There may be many explanations. Our job is to find out which one matter.

What do people do to remain cognitively healthy in their later years? One way to find out is to look retrospectively at the practices of healthy seniors. Find out what they eat, which medicines or health supplements they take, and how they run their lives. This kind of anecdotal information has been collected over the years and has led to the following widespread consensus: What works is a Mediterranean-style low fat diet, supplemented by selective vitamins, medicines that control blood pressure and blood lipids, and, equally important, actively engaging in both physical and mental activities. In other words, living a healthy, active lifestyle.

Can We Train Ourselves To Be Smarter Than We Are?

A billion-dollar brain training industry says yes, but not everyone agrees.

Is it possible for adults, even the very elderly, to improve their mental abilities? To stop forgetting what happened a few minutes ago or recall the title of the movie you saw the night before or learn faster and remember things longer? Lumosity, a web-based site first created almost two decades ago, promises to help you do just that. It reports to have millions of people who participate on line, and millions of dollars a year are spent to use their services. Widely advertised on many media, Lumosity offers on-line games that are designed to improve memory, increase attention span, enhance problem solving, and increase what they call speed of processing. Players are asked to solve challenging puzzles, and they are graded for speed and accuracy. Since these games are based on the way psychologists try to evaluate the mental status of people, it seems reasonable to expect that with repeated practice mental capacities should improve. Many studies appear to confirm that it does. A number of similar companies offer comparable services.

Brain-training companies typically offer players a chance to perform relatively simple skills in a limited range of contexts, yet they advertise themselves as dealing with a wide range of cognitive abilities. Some companies stand out for their efforts to document the scientific credibility of their claims, citing many studies by investigative psychologists who test their product. But relatively few of the studies were subjected to rigorous evaluations by scientists not involved in the study.

At this point we have to ask: What will we gain by spending 10 or 15 minutes several times a week at a keyboard studying colorful animations or dealing with progressively challenging number games? Will they have a lasting impact on our cognitive capacities and hopefully even lessen the likelihood of developing dementia? Indeed, the idea that changes in the brain could be achieved by training is truly revolutionary. But is it also true?

BRAIN GAMES ARE BOGUS declared Gareth Cook, a widely respected journalist, in a New Yorker article published in 2013[39]. Echoing the conclusions of a number of respected psychologists who specialize in brain development, he concluded that the claims made by Lumosity and others are largely unsubstantiated. A year later two groups of scientists waded in on the controversy. A group of seventy from around the world agreed that brain games do not provide a way to improve cognitive functioning or stave off cognitive decline, essentially in agreement with Gareth Cook.

This was quickly followed by a statement from an even larger group of scientists and practitioners who just as vehemently claimed that many studies did indeed confirm the benefit of brain training for a wide variety of cognitive problems and everyday activities. At this point one has to wonder: How could two groups of scientists who examine the same facts come to such conflicting views about the effectiveness of brain training?

To add salt to the wounds inflicted by skeptics, the Federal Trade Commission in 2016 fined Lumos Labs (the parent of Lumosity) two million dollars (reduced from a $50 million settlement) for false advertising claims. It was charged that inflated marketing claims misled the public by suggesting their games could stave off memory loss, dementia, and even Alzheimer's disease without providing any scientific evidence to back such claims. It is important to note that this judgement was based on what was perceived as misleading advertising not an assessment of the science behind brain training programs.

A major problem in the evaluation of any human health intervention, whether it be chemotherapy for cancer treatment or new ways to control heart disease is the complicating placebo effect. Scientists describe the placebo effect as a beneficial result produced by a drug or treatment that cannot be attributed to the properties of the placebo itself and must therefore be due to the patient's belief in the treatment. To register a new drug the FDA requires that a drug be subjected to double-blind randomized clinical trials in which the effects of the drug are compared with the effects of an inactive agent (the placebo). Both are given to carefully matched participants who serve as "controls". It is important that members of the control group believe they are being properly tested. Doubly blinded procedures are supposed to ensure that even the persons conducting the trial are unaware of who the control subjects are.

But it now appears that what works so well for evaluating drugs or medical and surgical procedures breaks down when psychological testing is involved. Evidently the type of person who agrees to participate in studies involving cognitive testing can unknowingly influence the outcome. This was discovered by psychologists at George Mason University when they decided to distribute two different posters throughout the campus to recruit volunteers to participate in a psychological experiment [40]. One poster stated up front that the study was designed to test a memory training program while the other poster only asked for participation in a study without specifying any specific goal. The goal of this experiment was to see whether a placebo effect could be due to the recruitment of individuals predisposed to believe that training of the brain was possible or even likely. The results were dramatic: Individuals assigned to the placebo group who self-selected by responding to the flyer emphasizing cognitive enhancement showed improvements after a single 1-hour session of cognitive training that was equal to a 5- to 10-point increase on a standard IQ test. Individuals who responded to the non-suggestive flyer showed no improvement.

We now realize that these results are not that surprising and confirm what earlier observers have noted. Individuals with strong beliefs in the malleability of intelligence have greater improvements in fluid intelligence tasks after memory training. These findings support those critics who suggest that placebo effects may underlie the positive outcomes seen in the cognitive-training studies that brain training companies used to support their claims. One has to agree that persuasive recruitment methods are likely to be a common problem in the brain-training industry.

There are several other significant failings of brain training games as they are currently practiced that must be acknowledged. The beneficial effects of training don't last very long, and those that do seem to be limited to the task that was being trained. There was little of what psychologists call the transfer effect, which is the capacity to extend what was acquired from the training of one test to improve the performance of other related tasks. Related to this was the claim that none of the tests have any measurable effects on one's ability to deal with real world problems.

Overall, the results show a fairly consistent pattern that on the face of it is not encouraging for people who hope to improve their mental capacities by the training programs now available. Improvements gained from these programs are hard to measure, and some even question whether the measurements that are used are valid. People who used programs that focused on speed of processing (how fast one can react) showed the largest gains both immediately and over time, but the benefits did not transfer to other mental activities that might have also benefited from an increase in mental processing speed. Moreover, the benefits in this group relative to the untrained group also diminished over time.

Yet if we look more closely at the criticisms of brain training we see a more nuanced picture. The question of durability--how long the improvements were maintained after training --is often cited as a major failing. In this regard one wonders whether the detractors protest too much. As described earlier, it is generally agreed that the adult brain is indeed capable of making structural changes in response to external input through the process called plasticity. Some like to compare plasticity changes in the brain to muscle development following exercise. Clearly muscles increase in size and strength in response to being stressed. But disuse atrophy, the loss of muscle mass, is a feature of inactive elderly people. Wouldn't one expect the brain to also lose its new-found capacities when the brain training stops?

Adam Gazzaley a neuroscientist at the University of California San Francisco has a different take on the brain training problem [41]. In his view most of the available commercial programs are not focusing on the right targets. He proposes that the human brain is confronted with multiple distractions that impose a destructive interference on our information processing systems. To deal with these distractions Gazzaley believes the brain needs to be challenged in ways that increase its ability to multitask and deal with multiple goals at the same time. His solution was to design a three-dimensional video game called NeuroRacer in which players use a hand-held controller to race a car on a video projection screen that shows a constantly changing road way. During the run signs begin to appear and disappear on part of the video screen. Some signs are important messages connected to the game, others are unrelated. The players learn to pay attention to the important signs and ignore the others. The goal is to keep the car running near the middle of the road and hit only the right signs. This is made more challenging by the game's computer that monitors the speed of the actions and adjusts the challenges to match the performance of the test taker. Gazzaley calls this a closed-loop system. The idea is that plasticity is stimulated by progressively increasing challenges. When this game was played by individuals of varying ages (ranging from 20 to 79), the youngest scored best in the initial testing, but older adults (60 to 85 years old) had a significant increase in their multi-tasking ability compared to active controls. Moreover, some trained elders achieved scores comparable to untrained 20-year olds, and the gains persisted for six months.

Despite the many caveats that dampen enthusiasm for most of the training programs now available, we should remain optimistic that more effective ways to train the brain to work better can eventually be achieved. The idea that the adult brain can be changed for the better is now a widely accepted fact. What remains to be determined is how we can implement it in a positive direction. Since the goals most people focus on are memory improvement, increased attention span and problem solving, attempts to achieve them have traditionally involved games that challenge the user to deal with increasingly complex visual situations as rapidly as possible. The challenge has been to devise games that deal with a specific mental capacity. What works for memory, such as repetition, might have less impact on attention span or problem solving. This is borne out by many studies that show that users only improve on the type of test they have been trained on.

So far, the most long-lasting improvement that has been achieved by a training program is the speed of one's mental reactions, often referred to as the speed of information processing. This is a critical process that undoubtedly plays a role in every activity that the brain performs. Processing speed surely contributes to everyday working memory, and, as was described in an earlier chapter, it is a function that is compromised in people with dementia. Figuring how to increase it for the elderly would go a long way to improving their mental health.

What is needed for successful and enduring brain training are computer-based programs that focus on specific targets that are based on sound scientific principles. The games must also be more creatively designed to entertain as well as inform. Ideally, users should regard them as pleasurable activities rather than boring burdens. It now seems clear that in order to benefit the elderly, training will have to be progressively challenging and on-going to generate long-standing benefits. Remember, brain plasticity can go in both directions.

What musicians have taught us about the brain

The pinky, the smallest finger of the hand, has a story to tell. Of all the fingers of the hand the pinky is least involved in our daily activities. But this is not the case for those who are trained classical pianists. People who spend a lifetime playing chords and practicing scales involve their pinkies in every activity. Studies of the brains of such people reveal that the parts of the brain that control pinky movements are significantly larger than in the brains of people who are not lifelong pianists.[42.] This remarkable finding indicates that repeated use of pinkies causes the part of the brain that control them to grow larger, and this applies to adults as well as young people. This is a remarkable example of the ability of the brain to grow during a lifetime and shows that plasticity, usually recognized as increase in function also has a specific structural explanation. Similar structural changes have been seen in the brains of other musicians and the adaptations that their brains display are specific for the instrument being played.

The significance of these findings goes beyond simply the confirmation of brain plasticity. It also predicts the prospect of rejuvenating brains in later life. If individuals at any stage in their adult life begin to learn to play a musical instrument they have the possibility of rejuvenating their brains because of the multiple challenge involved. Following a musical score involves seeing, hearing, and playing the instrument all at the same time, multiple challenges that stimulate growth and development. Clinical studies of elderly people support this prospect. Individuals who frequently played a musical instrument were less likely to have developed dementia compared to those who did not play an instrument. This protective effect was said to be stronger than those of other cognitive activities such as reading, writing, or doing crossword puzzles.

We know that aging is a risk that is hardly preventable. But other chronic diseases of the elderly are preventable, and some forms of dementia should be one of them. Major reductions in cardio-vascular disease have been achieved by changes in lifestyle, diet, physical exercise, and medications. In some cases, reductions by half have been achieved. Damage to the blood vessels of the brain should be similarly reduced by the same preventive measures. There is abundant evidence that an inactive mind is as susceptible to loss as inactive muscle.

Exercising the mind in appropriate ways may be the most effective way to keep the brain young.

Why such limited progress?

Why has there been such limited progress in the understanding of Alzheimer's disease? No doubt much has been learned since amyloid was re-discovered in 1984, yet one has to ask, why more than 30 years later, do we know so little about how to deal with the dementia problem? It is clearly a major health problem in many countries throughout the world and is predicted to increase in aging human populations. Factoring in immense human suffering and the prospects of bankrupting the healthcare system in the United States, reasonable people are entitled to ask: what have the National Institutes of Health, healthcare-related industries, and the scientific community been doing about it?

Alzheimer's discovery of plaques and tangles in the brain of a German woman who suffered all the complications of dementia first reported in 1904 was an important starting point since before that finding there was no specific target that can be considered the cause of such a complicated disease. This discovery went largely unnoticed until 80 years later when in 1984 three different research groups discovered the gene that was responsible for the amyloid protein. Finally, a specific target was identified that could be implicated as the cause of the plaques and tangles. The fact that these abnormal protein deposits were found in the hippocampus of the brain proved to be a crucial link between them and memory loss, since the fateful operation of H.M. in 1953 revealed that this was a major site for human memory.

The discovery of the amyloid gene was a major breakthrough since the experimental tools that DNA studies provide generated a wave of experimental studies in an attempt to link the amyloid proteins with brain damage. But unraveling the mystery of amyloid has proved to be a daunting challenge, and to this day it is still uncertain how these abnormal proteins cause brain damage although their presence in the late stages of the disease indicates that they are part of the problem.

The first FDA approved drug for dementia that appeared in the early 1990s was a drug designed to restore the ability of brain cells to talk to each other by providing a chemical that mimicked the natural signals. The first compound developed proved to be too toxic, but more recent varieties including Aricept are now in wide use. As stated earlier, it is truly remarkable that the most widely used FDA-approved drug for Alzheimer's dementia now available is one that was first developed nearly 30 years ago.

The bold attempt to remove amyloid from the brains of afflicted people by vaccinating them (which we now call immunotherapy) that began in 2000 involved a treatment that has been successful against many diseases and is still under intense development, as described earlier, but it still remains as the most promising form of treatment that may be on the horizon.

If one wonders why so few new discoveries have been achieved during the last two decades, the following chart provides a revealing answer.

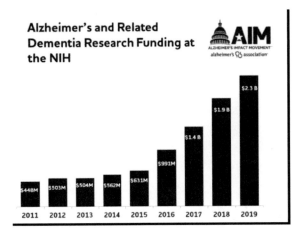

Of the billions of dollars the United States Congress awarded to the National Institutes of Health every year during the past decade, a remarkably small fraction was devoted to research on dementia and related diseases before 2016. During this period other major health problems, cancer, heart disease, and AIDS enjoyed multi-billion-dollar allocations. Put simply, before 2016 there was not enough financial support to maintain the level of research activity needed to study such a complicated problem as Alzheimer's disease. This changed dramatically in 2018, with the following announcement:

NIH is expected to spend $2.3 billion on Alzheimer's research in 2019. Clearly a number of factors influenced the decision-makers:

- A National Institute of Aging (NIA) funded study declared that Alzheimer's is the most expensive disease in the United States.

- The cost of caring for people with Alzheimer's disease annually is estimated to exceed $200 billion, with one hundred fifty billion paid for by Medicare and Medicaid.

- Dementia-related and social care costs are more than cancer and heart disease combined.

- If nothing is done to reduce its prevalence, it is estimated that over the next 40 years caring for people with Alzheimer's will cost the country $25 trillion with nearly 60% of that borne by Medicare.

The chart below predicts the future.

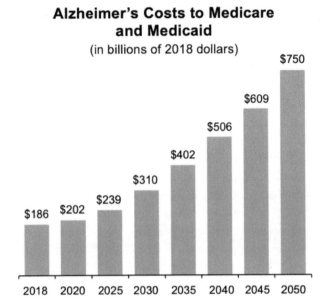

Alzheimer's Costs to Medicare and Medicaid
(in billions of 2018 dollars)

In addition to funds to support research provided by the National Institutes of Health and a number of nonprofit institutions such as the Alzheimer's Association, the pharmaceutical industry has also invested billions of dollars in an attempt to treat the amyloid component of dementia, as described earlier.

But there are other reasons why research on dementia lagged behind the other major health problems. Study of the human brain is a lot more challenging than studying any other organ. Take the simplest problem. The ability to biopsy the brain was and still is practically impossible. Before modern brain scanning technology was developed (in the early 2000s) Alzheimer's disease could only be diagnosed by autopsy. This meant that the diagnosis was based on clinical signs and symptoms that were often difficult to interpret.

The inability to diagnose the cause of dementia with any degree of certainty made it difficult to test potential therapies since the physicians never knew what the patients they treated were really suffering from. Every conceivable dietary component was either praised for its utility or damned for its complicity. Similarly, attempts to implicate all kinds of exposures to punitive brain toxins were made that could not be refuted.

Probably the biggest hurdle to productive research on dementia has been the lack of a suitable experimental animal model. Historically, progress in understanding human diseases has been based on the ability of scientists to create a pathological process in experimental animals that mimics a human disease. Cancer producing substances, called carcinogens, were first identified in animals, confirming their connection to many human cancers, and animals still represent the first step in the evaluation of anti-cancer drugs.

Imagine the excitement in the late 1990s when AD investigators announced that they had created mice that develop amyloid deposits in their brains which were considered to mimic the human problem. Through clever genetic manipulations, too technical to describe here, genes related to amyloid production were inserted into mouse brain cells and over time large amounts of amyloid accumulated in their brains that many investigators felt was similar to if not identical to that found in human Alzheimer's dementia. Was this the long sought-after animal model to study the development of dementia that could serve as a practical way to evaluate both new therapies and possibly even preventive measures? Many AD investigators thought so, and some still do, but so far, the potential of this approach has yet to be fully realized. Animals treated in this way do indeed accumulate large amounts of amyloid proteins in their brains, but the amount of actual damage to their brains is minimal with little convincing evidence that they suffer mental impairments comparable to humans.

The increase in funding that the United States Congress recently allocated to dementia research should have a major impact on many aspects of dementia research, not least the prospect of enlisting large numbers of new investigators into the field. The 1971 National Cancer Act did just that for the cancer field. The significant increase in research support for cancer research that was allocated by Congress convinced many basic scientists to shift their attention to the cancer field with very impressive results. Many new approaches to the treatment of cancers have been developed since then, and on the basis of what has already been achieved we can confidently predict that most cancers will be treatable chronic diseases. One hopes that an influx of qualified scientists into the Alzheimer's field will have a similar impact.

What I would do as a caretaker today

My wife's problems began more than four decades ago when little was known about this disease even by experts in the field. Although an active scientist I was as uninformed as any other caregiver. If I were a potential caregiver today my first impulse would be to seek the guidance of physicians in academic medical centers who specialize in dementia care and are aware of the emerging ways to evaluate cognitive impairments. Such analyses would begin with a thorough clinical evaluation that would include a number of different psychological tests that should be done by professionals in the dementia field.

Clinical evaluations can be informative as a necessary first step, but they must be backed up by specific laboratory-based tests, and first on the list would be the search for evidence of Alzheimer's disease. At the present time there are specific tests that address this question that are all based on the idea that the amyloid deposits might be the basis of her disease. The most direct way to measure amyloid deposits in the brain is to examine the fluid that surrounds it, called cerebrospinal fluid (CSF). This can be obtained by a relatively simple spinal tap, in which small amounts of CSF are removed and tested for the presence of specific types of amyloid peptides and for peptides related to the tau protein. These are highly specialized tests that must be carried out by qualified laboratories.

Abnormal levels of these peptides are presumptive evidence of amyloid deposits in the brain, but they're not definitive evidence of dementia. Fortunately, as described earlier, we now have extremely effective ways to scan the brains of living people to see whether they have amyloid and tau accumulations. A positive spinal tap along with positive brain scan would in most cases confirm the clinical impression that the patient suffers from a disease that we call Alzheimer's dementia. But this is not the whole story. A significant number of people in their mid-50s and older also have positive amyloid brain scans but are clinically asymptomatic. At this point I would not consider an expensive brain scan for Sally until we knew what we wanted to do with the information.

The most meaningful genetic test now available would be to see whether she has the ApoE 4 gene, that increases one's susceptibility to develop the disease. Her ApoE status will be particularly relevant since both her uncle and father died of early cardiovascular disease. Sally never had any symptoms of active heart disease, but vascular damage is definitely a factor in the pathogenesis of dementia.

What to do next is problematic. Drugs called Aricept and Namenda are believed by many to relieve the symptoms of the earliest stages of dementia, even though it is generally recognized that they do not influence the progression of disease. Unless her physicians felt strongly about it, my inclination would be to avoid both medications.

There is little doubt that accumulations of amyloid and tau are part of the problem, but not all AD investigators are convinced that they are involved in the early stages of the disease, a view I share. Nevertheless, it would be a mistake to ignore the possibility that amyloid deposits might be contributing factors. As described earlier, the ways to deal with potentially toxic amyloid deposits are still in the experimental phase. The most promising are chemical inhibitors that block the enzymes that create the amyloid peptides. These agents, called beta secretase inhibitors, are being developed by several pharmaceutical companies with early promising results. Compounds now available are able to reduce the load of amyloid in the brain, but the ones that have been developed so far have unacceptable side effects. If a safe FDA approved drug becomes available, I would consider enrolling Sally in an appropriate clinical trial.

Flushing amyloid out of the brain with antibodies, is another option that is under development by multiple pharmaceutical companies who are spending billions of dollars to create them as described earlier. After years of clinical trials their ability to make a meaningful impact on the progression of the disease is still in question. I would wait to see the outcome of these trials before considering such a treatment for Sally.

Can the progression of dementia be arrested?

How realistic is it to block the progression of existing disease? The answer is more positive than many people realize. Two factors support this optimism. Contrary to popular misconceptions, the actual incidence of Alzheimer's related dementia has been decreasing over the last decade. Evidently fewer people are developing the disease either because their exposure to pathogenic factors is decreasing, or, perhaps more likely, they have developed protective mechanisms. As emphasized earlier, there is no one single cause of dementia that has to be dealt with. Instead it seems that many potentially pathogenic factors might be acting incrementally over time and in their aggregate result in clinical dementia. Some may be more pathogenic than others, and if the most pathogenic ones are identified, dealing with them could be a big factor in reducing progression. In fact, there are at least a dozen identifiable factors that have the potential to contribute to disease development or related symptoms. Six involve diet and related metabolic problems and factors that might contribute to cardiovascular disease. Since we now realize that cardiovascular disease and dementia share many common properties, it is not unreasonable to suspect that the same factors that cause one contribute to the other.

- Diet
- Diabetes
- Obesity
- hypercholesterolemia
- Mid-life hypertension
- Smoking

The virtues of a Mediterranean diet have been described in great detail and are easily achieved by most people. Problems of metabolic dysfunction such as diabetes, obesity, and hypercholesterolemia are not so easy to deal with. They along with midlife hypertension need the help of qualified internists who understand their significance for dementia. Cigarette smoking, the source of much human pathology, can only be dealt with by individual behavior changes. Fortunately, smoking is on the decline in the United States, but not necessarily elsewhere in the world. It's interesting that the decline in the incidence of dementia mentioned earlier is most likely a consequence of the healthier lifestyles and the decrease of smoking that has taken place over the last several decades.

Many of these factors might have a minimal effect but if any major one progresses over time it can contribute to significant clinical disease. The total sum of the damage would depend upon the number of these potential causes and the magnitude of the problems they create. This explains why a two-decade long incubation precedes the onset of symptoms and why mental impairments become progressively worse over time.

Another set of factors that might contribute to the development of dementia include lifestyle and personal choices. These include

- Educational attainment
- Physical inactivity
- Mental inactivity
- Hearing loss
- Social isolation
- Depression

The level of education clearly plays some role in the development of dementia in later life, but it will be hard for most adults to do something about it. However, there are many instances where adult schooling late in life appears to have some benefit.

A proven way to enhance one's cognitive abilities at any stage in life is to engage in physical exercise. It is important to emphasize that this activity must be both significant in terms of challenging the body and meaningful in terms of adopting lifelong commitments. It is hard to predict how much physical activity is needed and which type of activity, aerobic or physical training, will be most effective for a given individual.

While compensating for physical inactivity is important for maintaining a healthy mental status, dealing with the consequences of prolonged mental inactivity is even more critical for maintaining one's cognitive abilities. It ranks as one of the most important ways to help arrest the progression of dementia particularly in early stages. The protective value of intellectual activity depends upon brain plasticity. The ability of the brain to respond to challenges is well documented. Unfortunately, this potentially protective process is clearly reversible. Challenging the brain by increasing mental activity increases its cognitive capacities, but relaxing that effort for too long a period runs the risk of losing all the newly created gains.

Hearing loss, social isolation, and depression are common to elderly people, but whether they put people at risk for dementia is controversial. Dementia and hearing loss are both highly prevalent neurologic conditions in older adults, each having considerable impact on quality of life. Some epidemiological studies suggest that hearing loss is a risk factor for the development of dementia[43] but how it is pathogenic is still unclear. Being hard of hearing tends to isolate people from others, limiting conversation that leads to social isolation, and, as described below, being socially isolated has long been recognized as a risk factor for cognitive decline.

Depression is common at older ages and often accompanies many chronic diseases, and it is associated with greater risk for mortality, higher health care costs, and disability. Some studies have suggested that persons who experience depressive episodes are at an increased risk of developing dementia in later life, but a very large study with a 25 year follow-up found that even chronic/recurring depressive symptoms do not increase the risk of dementia[44].

Like depression, it is uncertain whether social isolation is a potential cause of dementia or a consequence of being mentally handicapped. Some researchers have suggested that having a range of social connections is an important aspect of successful ageing and is associated with lower mortality rates and better health outcomes.[45] They reason that a rich social life enhances one's cognitive reserve that might protect against poor cognitive function in later life.

A Perspective

Alzheimer's dementia is considered by many to be the most feared disease that confronts aging human populations. To some extent this is due to doomsday predictions of popular media which suggest that the majority of individuals in their mid-80s will suffer from this debilitating disease. These are out-of-date statistics that need revising since they fuel discouraging negative views. Our inability to understand why protein deposits of plaques and tangles accumulate in the brains of people and how they actually cause disease makes treatment options illusive, but these are obstacles that will eventually yield to more informed research.

Blood vessel damage, an alternative proposal to explain dementia, is an idea that is consistent with the discovery that cardiovascular health and cognitive capacity go hand-in-hand. While the evidence in support of this idea is mounting, our ability to deal with it has yet to be defined.

Largely unnoticed by the popular media and even by knowledgeable scientists is substantial evidence that the incidence of dementia is declining rather than increasing, even though the total number of cases continues to increase as populations age. The simplest and most encouraging explanations of this decrease are changes in lifestyle and other factors that promote protective forces that were not available to people born earlier than the last half-century. These encouraging results suggest that the pursuit of preventive measures to combat dementia is the most realistic near-term solution to this world-wide plague.

One hopes that the significant increase in government support voted by Congress will be wisely allocated. I vote for support of studies that will research ways to implement the most effective preventive measures that have been identified by studies of people who have successfully defied the consequences of aging. How do we challenge the adult brain to continue growing? What are the most effective ways to exercise the aging body? What we now know is based on correlations. We need well controlled prospective studies to verify them.

NOTES AND REFERENCES

1. Squire, LR Neuron (2009) 61;6-9 The Legacy of Patient H.M. for Neuroscience.

2. Buried deep within both sides of the of the temporal lobes are regions of the brain referred to as the hippocampus. This region of the brain contains collections of neurons that are involved with memory functions and other related activities. Damage to hippocampal regions can result in a form of amnesia that involves loss of the ability to form new memories. This connection was discovered when a surgical operation designed to relieve intractable epilepsy removed the hippocampal structures of a 27-year-old man named HM. HM's inability to create new memories showed for the first time that the hippocampal neurons play critical roles in certain aspects of memory.

3. Magnetic resonance imaging (MRI) is a diagnostic procedure used by doctors to create pictures of the brain and other organs. It uses powerful magnets, radio waves and computers to detect changes in the brain not seen by traditional x-rays. Its main drawback is that it is quite expensive.

4. Dementia is a general term that describes a group of related mental symptoms that affect our capacity to remember and reason. People who suffer from dementia experience increasing confusion, inability to concentrate, changes in behavior and personality, and in the most extreme cases, inability to do everyday tasks. The most prevalent form of dementia in the aging population is Alzheimer's disease, a specific form of

dementia that will be discussed in more detail in this book. Other forms of dementia include dementia with Parkinson's Disease, fronto-temporal dementia, and Creutzfeldt– Jacob disease.

5.   Much of our body is made up of protein molecules. These come in a variety of sizes and shapes and do many things. Some join together into long strands of material that become our bones and joints and are called collagens. Some act as catalysts, referred to as enzymes, and they are critical for normal cell metabolism. Protein molecules that are damaged lose their normal shapes (and function) and clump together into aggregates that under certain circumstances can become pathogenic. When Dr. Alzheimer discovered what appeared to be clumps of material in the brain of his famous patient, he thought they might be the cause of her disease. Since that time different protein aggregates have been associated with many human diseases. The dementia associated with Parkinson's disease is characterized by Lewy bodies which are protein aggregates of another protein molecule.

6.   Amyloid is a protein that was first discovered by a famous German pathologist, Rudolph Virchow, who mistakenly thought that it was starch-like material since it could be stained with iodine. He called it amyloid (amylum in Latin), only later was it found to be derived from a protein and the basis for the protein deposits that are a characteristic feature of Alzheimer's disease.

7.   Nerve cells (neurons) have processes called axons that can extend long distances and connect to neurons in different parts of the brain. To maintain their stability, they have tubular structures in their cytoplasm called microtubules that provide the structural support. The microtubules are further stabilized by another protein, called tau. When tau is defective it falls off the microtubules and aggregates together in the form of long tangle-like structures. These were first observed by Alzheimer who called them neurofibrillary tangles. It is not clear why tau

accumulates and why it leads to cognitive decline; some believe that it is more relevant to dementia than amyloid plaques.

8. For the past 10 years, evidence has been building that the risk of Alzheimer's is declining in high-income countries. Scientists led by David Weir and Kenneth Langa, University of Michigan, Ann Arbor, reported November 21 in JAMA Internal Medicine that between 2000 and 2012 the prevalence of dementia in the United States fell a stunning 24 percent among people older than 65. The data come from the Health and Retirement Study (HRS), which includes people from different racial and socioeconomic backgrounds. Alzforum 25 Nov 2016.

9. Squire, LR J Neurosci (2009) 29; 12711-12716 Memory and Brain Systems.

10. The cerebrum and its outer layer called the cerebral cortex are the most highly developed parts of the human brain that are involved in thinking, learning, and understanding language. They are composed of populations of neurons that are connected to each other through their axonal extensions. Because of the dense concentration of neurons, the cortex is often referred to as "gray matter". It is divided into four lobes (frontal, parietal, temporal, and occipital) and each is responsible for processing different types of mental activity. The parts of the cortex most involved with dementia are the frontal lobes which are involved in personality changes and speech, and temporal lobes responsible for memory and language.

11. The amyloid hypothesis, first advanced by John Hardy and others, proposes that the accumulation of amyloid peptides in the brain is the key event in Alzheimer's disease. Their accumulation as plaque-like structures is believed to set off a series of events that ultimately results in the death of brain cells and subsequent dementia. Many versions of this idea have been published over the years, but there are still serious doubts whether amyloid works alone to damage the brain.

12. George Glenner, working as a scientist at the United States National Institutes of Health, discovered that the fragments of a protein, called the amyloid precursor protein, accumulated in the brains of people with dementia. It was shown to be the material that created the plaques that Alzheimer's first described in 1904. Glenner's discovery was possible because of the many advances in protein chemistry that have been made since Alzheimer's time.

13. This refers to the fact that large protein molecules can be broken down into smaller fragments, called peptides, by specialized enzymes similar to the ones that our gastrointestinal tract uses to digest meat. These enzymes in the brain are called secretases and are used by neuronal cells to create the amyloid peptides. This process takes place on a daily basis and is why amyloid peptides can accumulate into high enough levels to cause them to aggregate.

14. Genes are parts of the DNA of our chromosomes that determine what kinds of protein molecules our cells make. Genes, like proteins, are made up of multiple small units called nucleotides, and it is the linear sequence of four different nucleotides that determines what a gene does. Mutations happen when one or more nucleotides are replaced by others, creating proteins that are different from the originals. The modified genes that have been found in people with dementia who have inherited them are referred to as amyloid mutations. Fortunately, they account for a small fraction of the people with dementia.

15. ApoE, short for Apolipoprotein E, is one of many proteins in the circulating blood that is involved in lipid metabolism. Like other lipoproteins, ApoE has been implicated in the development of cardiovascular disease. But more than two decades ago, Allen Roses, a neurologist at Duke University and his team discovered that the ApoE molecule has three different forms, and one called ApoE4 turned out to be the most important genetic risk factor for late onset Alzheimer's disease.

16. Investigators of the University of Pittsburgh discovered a remarkable chemical that has the unusual ability to stick tightly to amyloid when it is present inside the body. When this material (called PIB) is injected into the bloodstream of people, it homes to sites in the brain where amyloid peptides accumulate. By using a special form of brain scanning called positron emission temography (PET), PIB lights up sites of amyloid deposits. Since this could be done with living patients, no longer is it necessary to wait for an autopsy to confirm the presence of amyloid.

17. Genotoxic is a term used to identify chemicals that can damage the genetic information of a cell, principally its DNA. Genotoxic agents include physical damage caused by radiation or a wide variety of chemicals. The most lethal genotoxins are also carcinogenic and can cause a wide variety of human cancers.

18. Oxygen which makes up 22% of the air we breathe can be converted into highly reactive forms (referred to as ROS), such as hydrogen peroxide that can modify all types of biological molecules. Oxidized DNA can be mutated, as described above, and protein molecules can lose their functions. Reactive oxygens can come from many sources, including polluted air and cigarette smoking, but they are also produced by the body itself during normal metabolism.

19. Virk, SA, Eslick, GD J Occup Environ Med (2015) 57:893-6 Occupational Exposure to Aluminum and Alzheimer Disease: A Meta-Analysis.

20. Bartzokis, G. Neurobiol Aging (2011) 32;1341-71 Alzheimer's disease as homeostatic responses to age-related myelin breakdown

21. Inflammation is a reaction of small blood vessels to injury. Any part of the body that has blood vessels can suffer from inflammation. Even a mild scratch of the skin causes the smallest blood vessels to enlarge, a process called

vasodilatation. The enlarged vessels leak water into the tissues causing swelling at the site that quickly resolves unless the injury is prolonged. More severe injury, such as an infection with bacteria, initiates a cascade of reactions: White blood cells accumulate and migrate into the tissues in search of the offending agents and remove them by phagocytosis. Inflammatory reactions can also damage normal tissues to produce what are called auto-immune diseases that can attack the heart (rheumatic fever), joints (rheumatoid arthritis), and the kidney (lupus erythematosus). Some regard inflammation of the brain as an under-appreciated problem.

22. The acquired immunodeficiency syndrome (AIDS) is a life-threatening condition caused by the human immunodeficiency virus (HIV) that selectively damages the immune system. The inflammation that is produced can also damage the brain and spinal cord. Hong, S and Banks, WA (2015) Brain Behav. Immun 45;1-12 Role of the immune system in HIV-associated Neuroinflammation and Neurocognitive Implications.

23. Plasticity is the ability of the brain to change in response to new challenges that can occur throughout one's lifetime. Long lasting functional changes in the brain are created when we learn new things or develop specialized skills such as learning to play a musical instrument or a foreign language. This is sometimes referred to as re-wiring the brain by making new connections.

24. Snowdon DA, Kemper SJ, Mortimer JA, Greiner LH, Wekstein DR, Markesbery WR (1996) JAMA 275:528-32 Linguistic ability in early life and cognitive function and Alzheimer's disease in late life. Findings from the Nun Study

25. Snowdon DA. (1997) Gerontologist, 37(2):150-6. Aging and Alzheimer's disease: lessons from the Nun Study.

26. Atherosclerosis, a modern term for "hardening of the arteries", refers to damage to the walls of medium and large arteries that can result in blockage of blood flow and death of the tissues they nourish. This vessel damage leads to the formation of

plaque-like structures, called atheromas, that contain cholesterol crystals and fibrous tissue. Atherosclerotic damage to coronary arteries is the most common cause of heart attacks, but it is now realized that atherosclerosis also damages the blood vessels of the brain.

27. Neurotransmitters are highly specialized chemicals used by nerve cells to signal to each other. Examples of neurotransmitters are acetylcholine and dopamine, two chemicals that are widely used throughout the brain. Neurotransmitters are critical for effective synaptic function

28. Immune therapy is a type of biological treatment that uses white blood cells and organs and tissues of the lymph system to fight infections and other diseases. Proteins in the blood called antibodies help us fight infection by their ability to neutralize specific pathogens. The idea proposed by Schenk was to see if antibodies that react with amyloid could neutralize it and render it non-toxic

29. Garrison SR, Kolber, MR, Korownyk, CS, McCracken, RK, Heran, BS, and Allan, GM (2017) Cochrane Database Syst. Rev 8; CD011575 Blood pressure targets for hypertension in older adults

30. Guallar E, Stranges S, Mulrow C, Appel LJ, Miller ER 3rd. Ann Intern Med. (2013) 17;159(12):850-1. Enough is enough: Stop wasting money on vitamin and mineral supplements.

31. A typical 28-gram serving of a milk chocolate bar has about as much caffeine as a cup of decaffeinated coffee. By weight, dark chocolate has one to two times the amount of caffeine as coffee. "Caffeine Content of Food and Drugs". Nutrition Action Health Newsletter. Center for Science in the Public Interest. 1996

32. Panza F, Solfrizzi V, Barulli MR, Bonfiglio C, Guerra V, Osella A, Seripa D, Sabbà C, Pilotto A, Logroscino G. (2015) J Nutr Health Aging. ;19(3):313-28. Coffee, tea, and caffeine

consumption and prevention of late-life cognitive decline and dementia: a systematic review.

33. Mazzanti G, Di Giacomo S. (2016) Molecules. 17;21(9). Curcumin and Resveratrol in the Management of Cognitive Disorders: What is the Clinical Evidence?

34. Nelson KM, Dahlin JL, Bisson J, Graham J, Pauli GF, Walters MA. (2017) J Med Chem. 60(5):1620-1637 The Essential Medicinal Chemistry of Curcumin

35. Laws KR, Sweetnam H, Kondel TK. (2012) Hum Psychopharmacol. 27(6):527-33. Is Ginkgo biloba a cognitive enhancer in healthy individuals? A meta-analysis.

36. Gurley BJ, Yates CR, Markowitz JS. Clin Pharmacol Ther. 2018;104(3):470-483 Not Intended to Diagnose, Treat, Cure or Prevent Any Disease." 25 Years of Botanical Dietary Supplement Research and the Lessons Learned

37. Myokines are small protein molecules that are produced in muscles during exercise. When released into the blood they can affect the functions of many other tissues. This may be the way that vigorous exercise activates the brain by acting as growth promoting factors as well as increasing the blood supply

38. Shatil, E (2013) Front Aging Neurosci 5;8 Does combined cognitive training and physical activity training enhance cognitive abilities more than either alone?

39. Gareth Cook The New Yorker (April 5, 2013) BRAIN GAMES ARE BOGUS

40. Foroughi, CK Monfort, SS Paczynski, M, McKnight, PE, Greenwood, PM Proc Natl Acad Sci USA (2016) 113; 7470-4 Placebo effects in cognitive training

41. Mishra, J Anguera, JA Gazzaley, A (2016) Neuron 90; 214-8 Video Games for Neuro-Cognitive Optimization

42. Schlaug, G Prog Brain Res (2015) 217; 37-55 Musicians and music making as a model for the study of brain plasticity

43. Thomson RS, Auduong P, Miller AT, Gurgel RK. (2017) Laryngoscope Investig Otolaryngol. 16; 69-79. Hearing loss as a risk factor for dementia: A systematic review

44. Singh-Manoux A, Dugravot A, Fournier A, Abell J, Ebmeier K, Kivimäki M, Sabia S JAMA Psychiatry. (2017) 74(7):712-718 Trajectories of Depressive Symptoms Before Diagnosis of Dementia: A 28-Year Follow-up Study.

45. Evans IEM, Llewellyn DJ, Matthews FE, Woods RT, Brayne C, Clare L; CFAS-Wales research team. (2018) PLoS One. 17;13(8): Social isolation, cognitive reserve, and cognition in healthy older people.

INDEX

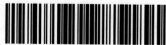

45814043R00046

Made in the USA
Middletown, DE
20 May 2019